HOME HEALTHCARE TELECOMMUNICATIONS

Technology to Improve Revenues

HOME
HEALTHCARE
TELECOMMUNICATIONS
Technology to Improve Revenues

RONALD J. PION, MD

STEVEN ALTMAN, DBA

LAURA HYATT, RN, BS, CCM

RONALD L. LINDER, EdD, MS

McGraw-Hill

New York   San Francisco   Washington, D.C.   Auckland   Bogotá
Caracas   Lisbon   London   Madrid   Mexico City   Milan
Montreal   New Delhi   San Juan   Singapore
Sydney   Tokyo   Toronto

Library of Congress Cataloging-in-Publication Data

Home healthcare telecommunications : technology to improve revenues /
    Ronald J. Pion . . . [et al.].
        p.   cm.
    Includes bibliographical references and index.
    ISBN 0-07-049449-5
    1. Home care services—Technological innovations.
    2. Telecommunication in medicine.   I. Pion, Ronald J.
    RA645.3.H655   1999
    362.1'4'028546—dc21   98–50620
                                                  CIP

McGraw-Hill

A Division of The McGraw·Hill Companies

1 2 3 4 5 6 7 8 9 0 1TGX / 1TGX 03 02 01 00 99

ISBN 0-07-049449-5

Printing and binding by TechniGraphix.

Cover Illustration by Steve Dininno.

This book was typeset using 11 point New Century Schoolbook.

This publication is designed to provide accurate and authoritative
information in regard to the subject matter covered. It is sold with the
understanding that neither the author nor the publisher is engaged in
rendering legal, accounting, or other professional service. If legal
advice or other expert assistance is required, the services of a
competent professional person should be sought.

    —From a Declaration of Principles jointly adopted by a Committee of
    the American Bar Association and a Committee of Publishers.

This book is dedicated to my family and friends whose love has authentic value. To the faculty and my colleagues of PKE 102 who continue to inspire; especially the committee of three: James Wilburn, PhD, David Hitchin, PhD, and James Martinoff, MD, PhD.

Laura Hyatt

To Sylvia (1900–1949) who would have preferred to have spent the last three months of her life at home; and to Paul (1905–1993) who might have been monitored more often at home. To all others whose quality of life and functional status can be assessed from a distance and remedied whenever possible via technology advancement and transfer.

Ron Pion

To Judy and Tyler, for their special brand of home care; to Mom and Dad, for staying on the leading edge with their support; and to all those who may benefit from the progressive developments described in this book.

Steven Altman

To my wife Kate for her continuous support throughout many evenings of solitude and my partner Rob Bonin for his encouragement; and a special thanks to Dr. Joy Cauffman, who as a co-worker opened my digital door many years ago on the SEARCH: A Link to Services project.

Ron Linder

C O N T E N T S

F O R E W O R D

There are few things more important than your health or the health of your loved ones. Usually this becomes more evident when someone's health is threatened. It is at these times that we rely heavily on the experience of professionals. We seek out those who can help us learn more about an illness and its possible treatment options. Medical professionals also require research data that can assist them in providing quality care.

Information and easy access to knowledge is power. Clinicians, healthcare administrators, and patients are entitled to it. This led me to create "Empower Health" which focuses on making healthcare information available to many audiences . . . anytime, anywhere. So, you can imagine my delight upon learning that the authors of *Home Healthcare Telecommunications* share my views. This book is a must read for anyone directly or indirectly involved with providing health-related services.

The elderly population is growing exponentially while simultaneously, advances in treating disease and its cost have led to a shift from hospital care to ambulatory services and home care. My colleagues explore the next logical step pointing out that as home care utilization increases, there will be a greater need to find more effective and efficient ways to communicate with patients and to manage their care at home. This will require that doctors and patients enter into a partnership to encourage greater responsibility for both prevention and treatment of illness.

It is exciting to contemplate the extent and depth of change to healthcare delivery that can be accomplished through the use of advanced telecommunication systems in the home. The dynamic evolution of the basic telephone permits large numbers of patients who are unable or resistant to the use of computers to benefit directly from Internet or Intranet based healthcare initiatives now being developed and implemented throughout the world. The newly emerging webphones will enable patients, for example, to access efficiently and download trusted medical information, participate in patient education and training programs, receive sophisticated day-to-day disease state management, monitor their medication compliance, and automatically re-order prescriptions and medical supplies.

To my knowledge, the authors are among the first to recognize the pivotal role that webphone-based technologies will play in the rapid advancement and escalation of healthcare communications. They clearly delineate fascinating new opportunities for gathering information for patients and healthcare providers that will result from the inevitable, widespread use of these new devices into the home.

Creating access to data from and to the home will be a most important driver of forward progress in the next century. *Home Healthcare Telecommunications* offers the reader pertinent information about using communications technologies as an important management strategy.

C. Everett Koop, MD
Former Surgeon General of the United States
Chairman, Empower Health Corporation

ACKNOWLEDGMENTS

This text was a team effort and as such the authors wish to acknowledge those persons who contributed their energies, time, resources, and support to this endeavor.

First we would like to express our appreciation to the publisher, McGraw-Hill, and especially to the editor, Kristine Rynne, who through it all was patient and gave positive direction.

Bellcore, Inc., offered support and intellectual capacity in the development of the book. Tom Moresco, Director of Advanced Services, was particularly instrumental, and we thank him and Bellcore for their help.

Pepperdine University provided access to information and guidance throughout this project, especially Arthur G. Linkletter, Board of Regents, and Chancellor Charles B. Runnels. The Graziadio School faculty and administration were generous with their knowledge, including Carl R. Terzian, Board of Visitors, Dean Otis W. Baskin, Associate Dean André van Niekerk, David Hitchin, PhD, James Martinoff, MD, PhD, Edward Sanford, PhD, Wayne Strom, PhD, Charles Fojtik, DBA, and James Wilburn, PhD, who is also Dean of the School of Public Policy. We thank them for their assistance.

Senior officers of companies were willing to give their time and share their perspectives about healthcare and technology. They deal with the realities of the industry on a daily basis, and we thank them for their contributions.

Our thanks to Edward D. Alston, Jr., a communications expert, who gave technical assistance during the writing of the book, and to Michael Villaire, who helped in the early stages of the book.

We would also like to acknowledge the following people for their efforts and support: Steve Adams, Pat Allen, Gale Alsen-Sebern, Rick Alvarez, Robin Amussen, Al Arakaki, Agnes Armstrong, Linda Bakken, Maureen Barry, Mark Beatty, Ed Boyer, Mary Cadogan, Betty Chan, Debra Cherry, Carol Corbett, Mike Corbett, Kevin Cornish, Frank Corrente, Linda Corrente, Maureen Cotter, Robert Craig, Michelle Crawley, Barit Darby, Connie Davis, J. Leonard Davis, MD, Paula Defusco, Dennis Diaz, Ollivier Dunrea, Rebecca Durham, John Elder, MD, Sandra Engle, Pat Evers, Paolo Fiorini, Debbie Fordham, Janet Frank, Susan Froberg, Rita Gallagher, Joe Gianguzzi, Harriet Gill, Richard Goka, MD, Roger Goodman, Amy Gross, Steven Gross, Toni Gross, Al Hackett, Howard Hamm, Mark Harling, Sunil Hegde, MD, Frankie Hershler, Joanne Holt, K. Hui, MD, Nadine Iba, Clair Jones, Sally Kaplan, Michael Kelly, Mike Kitzler, Joan Kraus, Leslie Larson, Judith Laughlin, David Leary, Linda Lee, John Li, Kim Lovetro, Christine MacDonell, Joe Martini, Richard McCarthy, Linda McCarthy, Joyce McClay, Denise McClinton, Beverly McGill, Barbara McIntyre, Pauline Merry, Roy Mitchell, the Montgomery Clan: Jane, Cliff, Marie, John, Sue, Peg, Paul, and Mark, Betsy Myers, Jason Myers, Judy Nuveau, Mort Olshan, Joane Ortiz, Lou Papastrat, Bonnie Parker, Ed Partis, Mary Partis, Richard Peck, John Perticone, Eli Pick, John Quinn, Bruno Raineri, Joyce Raineri, Terry Redderson, Emily Reese, Patti Robertson, MD, Dan Rosman, Tony Scaletta, Dave Scannell, Irv Schwartz, Selma Schwartz, Marie Scimeca, Barbara Smith, Suzanne Sonik, Audrey Stein, Ron Sympson, Tim Tillotson, Bill Timberlake, Karen Timberlake, Eric Toro, Mike Turner, Martin Valins, Charlene Vener, Jan Weaver, Margaret Weber, Nancy West, Neal Westermyer, Monika White, Bob Wilson, MD, Dave Wolf, Diana Wright, Alan Yellin, Carol Yellin, Diane Zajac, and Marty Zajac.

PREFACE

As we cross the threshold of a new millennium, we embark upon a journey to find solutions to current and future challenges. One such challenge is to provide healthcare that is cost-effective and compassionate. As a nation, we have traveled down this road before, but this time the difference is that we are armed with new tools. These tools are represented by sophisticated scientific knowledge about treatment, new business operations and management methodologies, and most significantly, the technology that will enable implementation.

Healthcare is undergoing reimbursement and regulatory changes that are creating problems for institutional providers, payers, consumers, and professionals. However, these difficulties that face us today will pale in comparison to those we will face tomorrow. This is because tomorrow's problems are compounded by two very significant factors.

First, the global nature of our lives. Once upon a time, healthcare was a community issue. If you became ill, you went to a doctor in town who treated you locally. Some elements of this are still true today; however, it is also true today that because of the ease of travel, diseases not only cross state lines, they cross continents. Organs for transplant are flown thousands of miles to get to their destination. Mega-mergers have created international corporations that may have healthcare operations in numerous countries, and the stocks of these companies might be traded on the Nikkei as easily as on Wall Street. These same companies are dependent upon revenues and financing in order to grow their business, and financing is affected by interest rates, which today, as never before, are impacted by the world economy.

Second, the shift in demographics is trending toward an aging population. Currently, there are more people over the age of 65 in America than the entire population of Canada. There are no signs of this trend slowing down; as a matter of fact, just the opposite is true. The "baby-boom" generation numbers 76 million, and they will begin reaching the age of 65 by the year 2011. Add to that an increased ability to diagnose, treat, and cure many diseases, and you have the ingredients to lengthen the average life-span. It is important to note that the United States is not alone in this dilemma; there are many countries that have their own version of baby-boomers. The good news is that many people will live longer. The bad news is that we are not prepared as a country or a world for such great numbers of people who will live longer but will also require healthcare.

One solution to the challenges of costs, care, and quality is to find ways for people to receive more care at home. This would reduce costs and is clearly the care site of choice. Ask yourself or your loved ones, "Where would you rather be cared for: in a hospital, nursing center, or at home?" In most cases, home is the clear preference. New innovations in technology allow for ease of information transfer and communication. The marriage of home healthcare and the new technology will encourage an expanded use of the home as a care site and therefore promote quality of life issues, and it just makes financial sense.

There are many potential opportunities for home healthcare. There are very real prospects for a delivery system that brings people back to the future. This future includes a care setting that regards a person's emotional, spiritual, and physical needs. It provides a vehicle whereby education and information can be exchanged and encourages appropriate self-management and responsibility. Through varied technological applications, we can create a healthcare delivery system that is effective and makes advantageous use of global research without jeopardizing intellectual properties or depleting financial resources.

The authors hope that this text offers the reader useful information for today and generates ideas for the challenges of tomorrow.

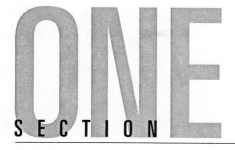

THE CHANGING CLIMATE OF HOME HEALTHCARE AND TECHNOLOGY

1 CHAPTER

Advancing Healthcare Communication

An Introduction

Healthcare throughout the world is experiencing a metamorphosis. This evolution is due to many factors, which are driving governments, providers, payers, and patients to revisit healthcare services, regulations, and reimbursement methodologies. Some of these factors are: the incidence and prevalence of disease and patient condition; research and development; changing reimbursement types and systems, including managed care; global economics; non-hospital capability; changing demographics and advances in healthcare technology.

The Congressional Budget Office estimates that U.S. healthcare expenditures rose to $1.09 trillion in 1997.[1] This number is expected to increase as millions of "baby-boomers" advance in years. This formidable group of 70 million people transformed the course of America, the most powerful nation in the world, ending the battle in Vietnam, and this same demographic group will fuel economic growth . This group will surely become the "change-champions," affecting nearly every industry in the third millennium.

It is our global responsibility to care for our communities in ways that are the most effective and efficient. Advances in communication technologies offer opportunities to employ these mechanisms in many areas including healthcare.

The need for information is critical to providing quality healthcare. One definition of communication is, the imparting, conveying, or exchange of ideas and knowledge. What affects the quality of our lives more than our health and often requires an exchange of information and knowledge? Telecommunications can provide the vehicle for such an exchange.

Technology is changing as rapidly as the field of healthcare. In addition to providing communication of information that is critical to recovery, telecommunications can deliver data rapidly. In healthcare, as in any business, time is money.

TEXT PURPOSE AND STRUCTURE

Amidst all of the changes taking place in the healthcare system, the inevitable question is why enter into or remain in the healthcare industry? The authors of this book would respond by asking, would you rather be part of an industry that is static or one that is fluid? The answer, of course, is one that is fluid because it encourages creativity. It invites leaders to come forward and create opportunities.

This book is about challenges and opportunities. As consumers and current economic conditions demand that the healthcare industry moves toward more home and ambulatory care, the challenge is how those services can be provided more efficiently. The idea of marrying the science of medicine and telecommunications presents an opportunity to increase effectiveness and decrease costs without compromising quality.

The purpose of this book is to familiarize the reader with salient information about healthcare, especially home healthcare and the effective use and availability of various forms of telecommunications. The following is a brief description of what is contained in each chapter.

Section One: The Changing Climate of Home Healthcare and Technology

Chapter 1: Advancing Healthcare Communication—An introduction addressing the importance and the purpose of the book and a brief description of each chapter. A discussion of the current status and direction of the healthcare industry, with an emphasis on home healthcare services.

Chapter 2: The Digital Emergence—The evolution and utilization of digital telecommunication is expanded upon along with its important role in medicine.

Chapter 3: The Business of Home Healthcare—An explanation of the changing nature of the healthcare industry in general with an eye on home care. Economic concerns are also addressed.

Section Two: Advances in Technology

Chapter 4: Telecommunications in the Home—An overview of technology currently available for use in home healthcare today. A review of data suggests success in reducing the costs of providing care.

Chapter 5: The New Screen Telephone—Equipment, education, and training are discussed. Segments of interviews with telecommunications manufacturers are also presented.

Chapter 6: The Telecommunications Industry and Healthcare—A dialogue about support services that may be necessary or advantageous and provides answers to frequently asked questions, such as those regarding costs.

Section Three: Beyond the Year 2000

Chapter 7: Future Challenges—Opportunities for healthcare providers and those who supply the industry are addressed. Strategies are also suggested to respond to challenges and create opportunities.

Chapter 8: The Age of Information Transfer (IT)—A look at what health-care in the year 2025 might look like. Projections regarding how home healthcare and ambulatory services will be delivered.

HEALTHCARE AND TELECOMMUNICATIONS—AN ABBREVIATED HISTORY OF PARALLEL TIMELINES

1840–1850

Healthcare

Medical convention is held in New York which later becomes the American Medical Association (AMA).

Telecommunications

Samuel Morse develops the Morse Code.

1850–1860

Healthcare

Uniform statistical research is gathered on causes of death and reported at an international conference.

Telecommunications

The telegraph expands across countries called the sea cable between England and France.

1860–1870

Healthcare

Major manufacturers, railroads, and mining corporations employ "company doctors." Medicine takes on greater social status and begins to be perceived as a science through the development of antiseptics, anesthesia, vaccines and the use of diagnostics.

Telecommunications

Johann Phillip Reis, a German teacher, invents the telephone.

1870–1880

Healthcare

Hospitals are licensed by states and begin to deliver more sophisticated medical services.

Telecommunications

Elisha Gray and Alexander Graham Bell acquire patents for the telephone.

1880–1900

Healthcare

Germany establishes the first national system of insurance.

The Mayo Clinic is established.

Formal training for nurses is instituted.

Telecommunications

Punched cards store data in U.S. for processing the census.

Dial telephones come into use.

Marconi sends signals over two miles by wireless transmission.

1900–1910

Healthcare

The AMA's Council on Chemistry and Pharmaceuticals gives MDs control of medications.

The first heart transplant is performed at the University of Chicago on a dog.

Prepaid medical care gets the nod from mutual benefit societies.

Telecommunications

The rectifier and triode usher in the electronic age.

1910–1920

Healthcare

Physicians begin to affiliate with hospitals.

Workers Compensation Laws are adopted by states.

Telecommunications

The AM Transmitter is developed.

1920–1930

Healthcare

Blue Cross adopts payment plans for hospitalization.

The AMA endorses routine physicals.

Telecommunications

The commercialization of broadcasting stations begins.

FM is developed.

1930–1940

Healthcare

The Social Security Act is passed.

More insurance companies begin to offer medical/hospital health plans.

Telecommunications

The first electronic transmission of television images takes place.

Multi-wire coaxial cables are developed.

1940–1950

Healthcare

Unions begin to negotiate for health benefits as a part of compensation under the Taft-Hartley Act.

The Hill-Burton Act makes federal matching funds available to hospitals.

Telecommunications

The development of printed circuit board eases the placement of components.

1950–1960

Healthcare

The nation's largest employees purchasing group is formed, called the Federal Employees Health Benefits Program.

Telecommunications

Aiken develops the electromagnetic computer.

Transistor radio and stereo recording are developed.

1960–1970

Healthcare

The physician coding system is introduced.

Medicare and Medicaid Systems are established.

Telecommunications

The first communications satellites are launched.

1970–1980

Healthcare

The Washington Business Group on Health is formed.

The HMO Act is introduced.

Telecommunications

Cable TV begins in the U.S.

Xerox introduces the first photocopier to the marketplace.

The programmable calculator and performance printer are developed.

The Japanese firm Matsushita patents liquid crystals for TV.

1980–1990

Healthcare

Health Care Financing Administration (HCFA) develops Diagnosis Related Groups (DRGs).

The Uniform Hospital Discharge Data Set (UHDDS) is created.

COBRA employee coverage takes effect.

HCFA publishes hospital mortality rates.

Telecommunications

The Hospital Satellite Network is formed.

Personal computers become prolific.

Compact discs, floppy discs, satellite navigation, videotext, and the Integrated Services Digital Network (ISDN) are developed.

1990–Present

Healthcare

The popularization of telemedicine occurs.

Competitive HMO contracts drives down reimbursement costs and lengths of stays in hospitals.

The HEDIS data set is introduced.

The first Wall Street conference on publicly traded physician groups is held.

The American Association of Retired Persons endorses HMOs for its membership.

Medicare risk plans expand and enrollment increases.

The Balanced Budget Act (BBA) is passed, and as a result, the Prospective Payment System (PPS) becomes inevitable.

Merger-mania takes over the healthcare industry.

HMOs begin to fall out of favor with consumers.

HCFA escalates its investigations of healthcare providers and institutions through Operation Restore Trust (ORT).

Cloning and gene therapy become a reality.

Designer drugs are developed to fight resistant bacteria and new diseases.

Consumers take a greater interest in health and fitness.

Telecommunications

Electronic media and mobile communications flourish.

The Internet phone is introduced in the marketplace.

The World Wide Web becomes one of the preferred places of commerce.

The Pentium Processor chip becomes the industry standard.

Broad wide bands, fiber optics, and ISDN make it possible to communicate in real time.

Information becomes available on demand.

THE CHANGING HOME HEALTHCARE INDUSTRY

The healthcare industry is comprised of a variety of professionals, institutional providers, payer sources, manufacturers, and suppliers of goods and services. Currently it is an industry in flux due to a number of factors. Economics appears to be the main instigator of these changes. The recent financial climate has caused mergers, buy-outs, unlikely alliances, and reorganizations in all areas of the healthcare industry.

This volatile state has created a new set of challenges and opportunities. It has also given rise to a new generation of medical business that introduced a daunting list of acronyms such as HMOs, PPOs, IPAs, MSOs, PSOs, HPICs, PHOs. ISNs, and IDS, just to name a few. Recent advances in technologies and pharmaceuticals that diagnose and treat disease are being developed faster than the Food and Drug Administration can approve them and in such volume that nurses and physicians are often unable to assimilate the vast amounts of information necessary to utilize them effectively.

In order to better understand the enormity of the healthcare industry, it is important to first have an understanding of some of its components. Those elements that offer direct clinical services might best be listed in order of the number and type of acuity of services available (Figure 1–1). The highest level and volume of acuity of services are provided by the organizations listed at the top of the columns with those offering a lesser volume of acute services listed at the bottom of the column.

High acuity services are often distinguished by the cost of providing that service. For example, acute care hospitals operate emergency rooms that require 24 hour licensed professionals, supplies, and equipment. This is a very expensive proposition which must be factored into the acute care hospital's overhead.

As a rule, the greater the volume of increased acuity of services delivered, the higher the costs. Following this line of reasoning, it is no wonder that there is an interest in moving as many healthcare services as possible toward home and ambulatory care.

Therefore, opportunities exist for those who are presently employed in home and ambulatory services or are interested in developing such services. It makes good economic sense, plus it promotes quality of life because most consumer surveys indicate a preference for home care versus institutional care.

FIGURE 1–1

INSTITUTIONAL	AMBULATORY
Acute Care Hospital	Outpatient Surgery Center
Acute Long Term Care Hospital	Specialty Treatment Centers (e.g., Dialysis or Infusion)
Specialty Hospital/Program	
Post-Acute Care Facility	Outpatient Facilities, e.g., Rehab
Skilled Nursing Facility	Home Healthcare
Nursing Home	Day Treatment Programs
Intermediate Care Facility	Diagnostic Centers
Assisted Living Facility	Physician Offices

The lists are ordered downward with highest acuity of services provided by those at the top of the list. Those entities listed in the left column generally offer an increased intensity of higher acuity services than those in the right column, and they incur greater costs partly as a result of operating 24 hours a day. It is important to note that in some cases high acuity services may also be provided by those organizations in the right column or further down the list.

CURRENT HOME HEALTHCARE INDUSTRY STATUS

The number of home healthcare agencies has nearly tripled during the decade representing the late eighties into the late nineties. Specifically, there were over 5,250 agencies operating in 1986 compared with 14,670 agencies in 1996. Home care chains accounted for 32.4% of agencies in 1996, 11.6% were government agencies, and independent agencies represented 47.8%.

The top 40 home care chains operated 3,649 offices in 1996 and managed nearly one quarter of all home care offices, with ten of these chains maintaining offices in more than 25 states. Twenty-nine of the largest chains were for-profit corporations in 1996, accounting for 26.4% of all home care agencies. The independent for-profit agencies totaled 29.8% of the industry, while 18% of the agencies were organized as independent not-for-profit. In 1996, 52.7% of home care agencies were Medicare-certified, resulting in a gain of over 10% from the preceding year.

Home care agencies employed an average of approximately 46 full-time-equivalent workers per agency in 1996. In the same year the top chains employed about 146,000 workers. Based on the number of agencies in the United States (14,670) and the average number of full-time-equivalencies per agency (45.63), the home healthcare industry was estimated to have 669,392 employees in 1996.

The types of employees that work for home care agencies are physicians, registered nurses (RNs), licensed vocational nurses (LVNs), licensed practical nurses (LPNs), physical therapists, occupational therapists, speech and language pathologists, case managers, respiratory therapists, dieticians, personal care aides, administrators, managers, and clerical, legal, informational, and financial personnel.

Home healthcare agencies reduced their full-time staffs in 1996 from the previous year's levels. This reduction in force was the result of mergers and acquisitions, and the need to reorganize to keep pace with lower reimbursement amounts. Medicare-certified home care agencies provided an average 656 visits per week, which was about 1.5 times greater than those of non-certified agencies, which averaged 435 visits per week in 1996. In the same year, registered nurses provided an average of 176 home care visits per agency per week and licensed practical nurses averaged 100 visits per agency per week, while home healthcare aides averaged 277 visits per agency per week.

Chronically ill patients comprised 44.6% of the patient population of home care agencies in 1996, which was an increase from 1995 levels. Government-owned agencies reported that over 53% of their patients had chronic illnesses. Patient's dependent upon wheelchairs in 1996, numbered 16.3%—almost three times as many as in 1994. Patients with AIDS represented 3.6% and those suffering from Alzheimer's Disease rose to 8.7% in 1996.

In 1996, home healthcare agencies reported a substantial increase in patients 75 years and older, accounting for 39.6% of their total patient population. The gender gap exists among home healthcare patients, with agencies indicating an average of 36.7% males and 63.3% females. Patients seen by home healthcare agencies for less than 30 days averaged 28.2% of the total patient population in 1996, while those receiving services for more than 30 days numbered 71.8% of this population.

In 1996, home healthcare agencies stated that 33.7% of their patients lived alone, 53.5% lived with a spouse or with family, and 11.8% were living with a friend. In addition, 26.6% were temporarily incapacitated while 7.2% were reported to be in the last six months of life.

Medicare payments accounted for two-thirds of agency revenues in 1996 at 65.2%. Medicaid represented 9.6%, while private insurance and self-pay was 13.6%. HMOs and PPOs averaged 5.6% of the accounts receivables in the same year. State and local government averaged 3.5% and bad debt amounted, on average, to 0.8%. Charitable contributions and other supplemental payments totaled approximately 1.7% in 1996.[2]

HOME HEALTHCARE TRENDS

Hospital occupancy rates are shrinking as patients are rerouted to less costly alternative sites of care. This has been a decade-long trend, in which the home and ambulatory care population has risen by 70%. Many of these patients who would have been hospitalized only ten years ago are now being redirected to home healthcare and a variety of ambulatory care sites, such as clinics, outpatient surgery and therapy centers.

Home healthcare is becoming a stronger force weighing in at projected revenues of $42 billion in 1997. This seemingly large number only represents a little over 4% of the entire amount of current healthcare expenditures. Healthcare experts along with Wall Street have predicted that this industry will account for over 10% of U.S. healthcare expenditures by the year 2005—that is, in less than half a decade. As remarkable as that number may be, the authors of this text would suggest that it should and most likely will be even more.

The reasons are simple. Given what we know today, home healthcare represents an environment that is effective for treating many kinds of illnesses and injuries. It allows for less cost prohibitive care than is provided when a patient is hospitalized. Most importantly, it is the consumer's first choice for a care-site. Think about it. In most cases, if you were asked whether you would rather stay at home or go to a hospital or nursing home, what would your answer be?

There are many signposts pointing the way to an increase in the use of home and ambulatory services. Hospital corporations are consolidating, and although many might have expected more closures to have occurred by now, this probably will happen over the next five years. The number of acute hospital bed days per thousand lives will continue to decrease across the country as the healthcare industry coupled with science finds new and less costly ways to deal with disease.

TELECOMMUNICATIONS AS A PLATFORM FOR HEALTHCARE EFFECTIVENESS

Telecommunications is one way in which we can improve upon the delivery of healthcare services in alternate sites of care. Some of the possible benefits of telecommunications are:

1. Promoting the use of primary, ambulatory, and community care through decision support and diagnostics by telecommunications technology

2. Creating community health and patient monitoring systems that provide data encouraging consumer responsibility and self-managed care

3. Developing international data banks that facilitate the referral and transfer process

4. Reducing redundancy and unnecessary duplication so that resources are shifted, from the more costly inpatient settings, when appropriate, to home and ambulatory sites

5. Significantly decreasing the lengthy waiting and travel time of professionals and patients caused by delays in communication

6. Increasing the efficiency of information exchange between clinicians and management to better administer healthcare

7. Improving financial arrangements through the use of electronic information

8. Facilitating care coordination and effective case management

9. Designing the strategic integration of service delivery

10. Standardizing practice, technologies, patient classification systems, and protocols through an international network

11. Providing a vehicle that enables consumers to gain access to information on demand, thereby creating a partnership for wellness

12. Supporting the development of an international healthcare communication infrastructure

13. Encouraging international research and development collaboration

14. Re-engineering cost to benefit strategies between purchasers and providers

15. Writing disease management programs based on data across continents

16. Creating immediate access to outcome information

17. Expanding existing knowledge and ideas about service integration

18. Promoting interactive clinical alliances between health practitioners
19. Procuring critical data that is adaptive to context and need (for example, when monitoring local or regional epidemiological situations)
20. Increasing access to practitioners
21. Improving the monitoring of medication compliance with links to pharmacists and pharmaceutical manufacturers
22. Encouraging ease of transferability and understanding of services across cultures
23. Reducing the time spent on licensing, surveys, accreditations, and credentialing by entering data prior to onsite visits
24. Building tele-training labs for clinicians, administrators, and patient teaching
25. Improving patient satisfaction and the quality of care through an informed collaborative community

"SHIFTING GEARS"

This is the short list of possibilities that exist through the use of telecommunications in healthcare. As with any new paradigm there are constraints. The most obvious one is that it is "new" and requires a shift in thinking and attitudes. It necessitates financing for research and development. It requires leadership that is committed and has a clear vision.

This shift demands that as a scientific community, we toss aside the shrouds of secrecy that have kept us from partnering with our patients or clients and our medical colleagues. In order for healthcare to advance to the next level and for the human race to truly embrace compassion, we must not be so arrogant as to believe that there is any benefit to withholding the answers in the name of competition.

For all of the purists, the authors wish to acknowledge that they are not suggesting that telecommunications should replace doctors, nurses, or any other healthcare professional, but rather, that it should enhance their ability to perform at optimum levels. Two of the authors, after all, are clinicians.

There is no substitute for a face-to-face initial examination. It requires skill, knowledge, experience, person-to-person contact, and the ability to use of all of one's senses, and perhaps most importantly, one's intuition.

Other challenges are discussed in more depth in later chapters of this text. Strategies including strengths, weaknesses, and trends driving the changing landscape of the healthcare industry are also explored.

THE BUSINESS CONCEPT

In the home and ambulatory care arena as in every other area of the healthcare industry, developing consumer awareness and building product differentiation are important. This concept of value-added services takes on new meaning as reimbursement becomes standardized according to regional rates and competition rises to a different level.

Until recently, the healthcare industry has resisted viewing itself as a business. Hence, certain business concepts, such as brand or product management, which are taken for granted in most other industries, are in the healthcare industry, poorly understood, rarely discussed, and almost never implemented.

The "build it and they will come" philosophy began to slip away with the advent of the Omnibus Reconciliation Act (OBRA) and the proliferation of managed care in the 1980s and 1990s. The third millennium will bring a new set of challenges with the implementation of the Balanced Budget Act (BBA) and the introduction of the Prospective Payment System (PPS).

The Prospective Payment System, or PPS—its familiar acronym, will change the way in which healthcare organizations provide care and are reimbursed for services. It requires that, once again, providers must tighten their belts and find yet another way to reduce overhead in order to make a profit and, in some cases, just cover their costs. It also mandates the electronic transmittal of financial and clinical data.

Home care agencies and other ambulatory services will be required to submit more data, with new methodologies and under very strict time constraints. The data that is entered and sent electronically to HCFA will determine not only the amount of payment but also whether or not the provider organization will be reimbursed at all. The importance of having a responsive data system in addition to continuous training and monitoring of personnel becomes even more significant for the provider's future financial survival.

Case mix data along with outcome information will be crucial in collecting proper reimbursement and maintaining market position. Case management relies heavily on this type of input in order to operate effectively. Most healthcare entities have seen the wisdom of employing an experienced professional in this position to assist with assessment, coordination of services, and obtaining verification and authorization for payment. Telecommunications is an integral aspect of the agency's ability to interface with those purchasers who will expect even more information in the future.

MEETING THE STANDARD

Home healthcare agencies must undergo certification and accreditation in order to receive reimbursement from government agencies. This process is also necessary in order to secure most managed care contractual arrangements.

Most accrediting bodies, such as the Joint Commission on the Accreditation of Healthcare Organizations (JCAHO), and CARF—the Rehabilitation Accreditation Commission, require that the provider organization choose a system, and collect outcome data that has been input into that system for at least a year prior to the survey. This data is then used by the healthcare provider to benchmark themselves against other like organizations in an effort to demonstrate that they are providing care that measures up to a certain standard. Also, the provider is supposed to utilize the information as a means of managing the quality of care and/or to study specific treatment modalities that could be improved on. Once they have identified these areas, the provider is then expected to illustrate that a plan was implemented to improve care.

This is an important part of the survey process, and is often an area of weakness for organizations. It is doubtful whether providers can meet this accreditation standard without the use of telecommunications technology, especially given that most information that is gathered is then processed through a national data system.

CONCLUSION

This book contains useful information that has practical applications for professionals, providers, payers, and those that manufacture or supply equipment, products, and services to the healthcare industry. It also provides insights about ambulatory and home healthcare to those involved in technology and telecommunications who are interested in offering their products or services to healthcare organizations.

It is appropriate that healthcare is entering a new era of information and technology as we approach the third millennium. This text offers a glimpse into the expectations, challenges, and opportunities that will come as healthcare interacts with the technologies of telecommunications.

REFERENCES

1. The Congressional Budget Office: *The Economic and Budget Outlook*, Washington, D.C., 1997.
2. Roussel: *Managed Care Digest Series*, pp. 33–38, Kansas City, MO, 1997, SMG Marketing Group Inc.

2 CHAPTER

The Digital Emergence

Data, images, video, and audio can now be transformed into one common denominator: the bit. Bits are binary digits of "1s" and "0s" forming an electronic code that allow information to be stored, transmitted, and transformed back into their original state (e.g., a picture, graphic, music, or film clip). Digital technology makes use of bits to represent various forms of information. One of the most recognizable uses of digital technology is the computer.

The digital door is opening and many challenges await. The complexities that overlay the digital media business are technical, political, functional, territorial, financial, and difficult to overcome. Many telecommunication providers and users are frustrated and do not know which path to take in designing or selecting systems and applications. The positive aspects of digital technology include its quality, versatility, and potential transport speed and accessibility. The negative aspects include fragmentation of efforts in creating digital system standards, lack of support structures to deliver them, and high initial costs of their implementation.

For example, the television industry is about to introduce high definition television (HDTV)—the application of digital technology to television. There is still little consensus on technical standards, on what the public wants, and what is affordable. However, experts do believe that HDTV will ultimately win out once the technical specifications have been determined and consumers actually see a sharper television image. Nevertheless, analog and digital television are likely to coexist in the broadcasting industry for at least the next decade. Digital transmission to the home is a major emphasis of network providers and will most likely occur before digital televisions are widely available.

After reviewing many of the complexities associated with opening the "digital door" to home healthcare, a complete transition to digital technology may take much longer than desired. Like the television industry, home healthcare providers and consumers, with user terminals being equivalent to televisions, will probably have to live with a combination of analog, digital, and transitional terminal systems for some time.

This chapter identifies major benchmarks in the evolution of telecommunications, leading to a general discussion of its applications in home healthcare. The section in this chapter on digitizing healthcare introduces the use of integrated Home Health Telecommunications (HHT) and its related costs and benefits. The chapter concludes with a few HHT pathfinding hints to consider when searching for the right system.

Perhaps the biggest question addressed by this chapter is "How does one proceed after opening the digital door?"

EARLY TELECOMMUNICATION PATHWAYS

Major historical benchmarks in the transmission of information, in addition to those identified in Chapter One, have evolved in a variety of unusual and interesting ways over the centuries, as described in the following text.

1876–1892: Dial System Without Operator Assistance Is Introduced in the United States

The use of the telephone underwent a major expansion with the introduction of automated dialing systems, which reduced the need for thousands of operators and significantly decreased the time required for dialing. This made the telephone a highly private, instantaneous means of communication and established a new system of business and personal connections over time boundaries throughout the entire world. Switching technology helped establish the telephone as the major communication tool of the future.

1917–1957: The First Television Images Are Transmitted in Berlin

Much like the telephone, the introduction of television was another revolutionary addition to mass communication with an extraordinary potential for linking people and events worldwide. The early combination of the telephone and television enabled newscasters to bring live reports of world events into the living rooms of America. It would later become a highly effective means of bridging communication gaps between individuals and isolated events, subsequently leading to the development of vital medical diagnostic and educational applications. For example, the development of arthroscopy and endoscopy relied on the science and technology of the television.

1960–1985: The First Communication Satellite

While interest in using video technology to transfer information was growing in the 1960s, the introduction of communications satellites dramatically expanded broadcasting range and provided the foundation upon which new approaches to communication could be shared and tested. The capacity to provide live global video communication had long been awaited. It started with live one-way satellite transmissions of a television signal, with the ordinary telephone linking on-camera presenters with their viewers. The federal government and the National Aeronautics and Space Administration (NASA) took the lead in research and development. The Veterans Administration (VA) was the first large healthcare provider to experiment with live videoconferencing by satellite transmission. Initially, the major obstacle to its early success was the constant preemption of scheduled VA satellite time by various government agencies, such as the Department of Defense.

By the early 1980s, the Hospital Satellite Network (HSN) began transmitting live by satellite, providing 16 half-hour accredited professional education programs every month to its 1,000 subscribing hospitals, including the entire VA healthcare system. HSN became the largest single provider of professional education in the country's healthcare system during the late 1980s. Rural hospitals in particular benefited from these distance learning opportunities. In addition, live videoconferences on a variety of topics enabled healthcare providers to communicate by telephone with presenters during the actual telecasts. Unlike the VA's earlier experiences, no preemptions of transmission occurred. Many of these events involved intercontinental satellite linking of world leaders in healthcare.

1980s–Present: The Internet

Among the latest milestones in telecommunications are the computer and the establishment of the Internet. The Internet was developed in the late 1950s as an information network for the Defense Department. It then began to be used by universities for research, and in the 1990s, the Internet became an important network for businesses. Most recently, the Internet and the World Wide Web present an array of information never before available to the masses. The Internet also provides users with a range of services enabling interactive communication between individuals and groups over regular telephone lines. Due to the early creation of the telephone, which provided the essential network of wiring, the World Wide Web is today a reality, offering the capability to move data, images, video, and audio everywhere that telephone wiring exists.

By 1997, SEARCH: A Link to Services had established a computerized database of professional profiles, services rendered, second language capabilities, and payment options of physicians, dentists, psychologists, and social workers throughout all of Los Angeles County, California. Consumers simply had to call a local telephone number to obtain assistance through a computerized operator. Through this federally funded project, the first computerized database of healthcare providers for a major city in the United States was created. This system also pioneered the use of on-line updating of databases.

The underlying message of these four examples of telecommunication applications over a twenty-year span is the consistent, vital role played by the telephone and its two copper wires, which serve as the critical links to services that were never anticipated at the time the telephone was invented.

THE TELEPHONE

In 1877, the first permanent outdoor telephone wire reached a distance of three miles. One year later, calls could be switched over hundreds of miles. By 1879, subscribers were assigned telephone numbers because of a measles epidemic. A Massachusetts physician, concerned about replacement operators unfamiliar with the names of local subscribers, recommended a numeric system. A Kansas City undertaker who thought local telephone operators were sending his business elsewhere patented the first automatic dialing system in 1891.[1]

Party lines, requiring neighbors to share one line, were made available, particularly in rural areas, to lower the cost of telephone service. Ten million Bell System telephones were in service by 1918.[2] The technology was expanded and refined to the extent that the demand for telephones had surpassed the supply.

Since then, the telephone has promoted the worst and best of society. It has played a significant part in waging wars, expanding human conflict, and providing a conduit for criminal activity. On the positive side, the telephone has saved lives by creating access to emergency services, rapidly transmitting vital information, removing isolation among homebound individuals, promoting industrial growth, and improving the quality of life. In the midst of technological alienation, the telephone continues to be the ultimate compensatory invention that immediately brings people together with great ease. Furthermore, it continues to be the vital component of HHT.

THE TELEPHONE AND HOME HEALTHCARE

The true beginning of HHT was in the late 1870s, when the first telephone exchange connected over twenty local doctors with a community drugstore in Hartford, Connecticut. This led to the first telephone exchange and long-distance connections between Boston and New York City by 1884.[3]

One can only guess at the myriad contributions the telephone has made to healthcare delivery. The ability to reach a physician by telephone has dramatically reduced the human costs of health emergencies. Telephone links to the drugstores were rapidly expanded to include medical message centers, which provided a way for families to keep in contact with the doctor in the absence of office visits and house calls. By 1974, consumers could use the telephone to access brief recorded messages on various health topics.

We have come a long way in all aspects of life by way of the telephone. Historically, one might consider the invention of the telephone to be a major technological breakthrough in medicine. The telephone continues to be the most used telecommunications link throughout the world, with many local connections still made by a simple network of small copper wires.

TELEPHONE LINKS TO HOME HEALTHCARE

The home may well become the primary site of medical care (and all other settings may become alternate sites). Not only is the home the most humane environment for the delivery of care, it is most preferred by patients and families. Once reimbursement policies support managing the care of patients in the home, the use of communication technologies and related services will become even more essential and cost effective. Increasingly, patients can expect to receive more of their healthcare, when medically appropriate, in their homes rather than in institutions.

New technologies make it possible to establish a home-based "hospital" by providing two-way communication links for providing such forms of healthcare as infusions, dialysis, insulin therapy, respiratory services, blood glucose monitoring, home ventilators, and IVs. Healthcare providers can now use state-of-the-art technology to remotely monitor vital signs, diagnose and manage certain patients, resuscitate homebound cardiac arrest patients, monitor high-risk pregnancies, administer medications, and manage pain. Such healthcare services—brought to the home by the telephone alone—can revolutionize the roles of care providers and their patients.

One of the most effective areas of telephone use in healthcare is triage. Many outpatient clinics use telephone triage to maximize existing services and reduce unnecessary visits. Patients access the system or receive advice by telephone, rather than going to a facility as an unscheduled walk-in patient. The telephone triage system is designed to optimize care through the following benefits:

- Providing early assessment, proper referral, and effective scheduling of patients
- Relieving congestion in critical areas such as the ER and walk-in outpatient clinics
- Identifying certain patient healthcare and learning needs

If the triage nurse is uncertain about the disposition of the patient, other members of the provider team attending are queried for advice. To expedite an appointment, the triage nurse initiates by telephone the diagnostic work-up by ordering chest, limb or skull x-rays, EKGs, blood tests such as serum drug levels, routine urinalysis, and chemistry panels. This information is entered into the computer system, and a progress report is electronically produced and available by the patient's scheduled visit.

Through the use of Interactive Voice Response (IVR) systems, patients can now be screened by telephone, which is just as effective as a written questionnaire or personal interview. Follow-up and counseling, reminders, and interactive educational programs and services are among the most effective applications of the telephone in expanding home healthcare (Figure 2–1). The consumer merely calls from a touch-tone telephone and responds to a series of programmed questions by pressing the appropriate key designated for a given answer.

FIGURE 2–1

Effective Telephone Applications to Home Healthcare	
Alzheimer Disease	3
Appointment/Show Rates	2
Cardiac Care	1
Diabetic Foot Care	2
Tobacco Use Prevention	1
Immunization Rates	2, 3
Medication Compliance	2
Mammography Use	1
Osteoarthritis	1, 3
Problem Drinking	3
Emergency Department Visits	1
1, Follow-up/counseling; 2, reminders; 3, interactive.	

Source: E. Andrew Balas, et al: Electronic Communications With Patients, *JAMA* 278(no. 2), 1997, pp. 152–159.

Many of these systems require prolonged periods to complete a series of questions; however, the use of personal identification numbers (PINs) allows callers to leave the system and return later to complete the process. This approach has been used extensively in screening patients for participation in various self-management programs that include video and print support materials. The same IVR system is often used to assess patient outcomes, order self-management packages, and provide additional therapeutic support.

Many projects making use of the telephone have been conducted in an attempt to increase access to care and reduce the costs of delivering it. Most demonstration projects were directed by professionals at academic health centers, using the "hub-and-spoke" approach. They usually applied real-time technologies and focused on specialty consultations. Subsequently, demonstration projects rapidly spread to many areas, including cardiology, orthopedics, dermatology, psychiatry, oncology, renal dialysis, urology, trauma, and ophthalmology. The use of the telephone has also proven to be highly effective in managing certain types of emergency room visits. Pediatric emergencies, patients with urinary tract infections, and certain acute and chronic conditions all respond better with telephone follow-up and counseling. Benefits have also been observed for inpatient management following cardiac surgery, acute myocardial infarction (i.e., heart attack), smoking cessation, cholesterol management, length of recovery, adherence to routine screenings, medical compliance, and the management of osteoarthritis. Initially, few projects included HHT applications.

Telephone reminders improve compliance in medication use, preventive measures, fulfilling instructions, and keeping appointments. Significant improvements in foot care by diabetics and activities of daily living by osteoarthritis patients can be attributed in part to telephone reminders.[4]

The use of prerecorded telephone messages or instructions and informational programs and reminders have been expanded by touch-tone Interactive Voice Response (IVR) systems. Patients can access additional information simply by pressing certain numbers on their telephones. Appointments can now be made or changed using IVR systems. Knowledge about Alzheimer's disease, immunization visits, and medication adherence among elderly patients improved following the use of an IVR system. A question and answer format is one of many approaches used effectively in linking patients with appropriate information.

Touch-tone telephone IVR systems are being used to query patients at home about their chronic health problems and determine their eligibility for self-help interventions. In one program, patients qualifying through an IVR administered questionnaire are given a PIN number, and self-help educational videos and print materials on managing their chronic conditions are sent by mail. They are initially given an orientation video that prepares them for choosing from three self-management options: diet, sleep, and self-medication. After selecting one of these interventions, patients order their self-management materials by merely picking up their telephone and responding to another set of IVR questions. Patients use the same system to report their progress or order additional interventions for controlling their heartburn. Once again, the telephone provides for high touch interactive communication.

Capitated managed care systems have built-in economic re-wards for efficiency, particularly when offered quality-enhancing solutions to patient care challenges. The current trend toward in-tegrated care management systems, in which physicians assume the financial risk, should hasten the adoption of more efficient and cost-effective communication solutions, including the tele-phone, that address travel requirements, time limitations, dis-ease management costs, and quality of care issues.

What has made the transition to HHT so difficult is the lack of affordable communication links that meet the vast needs of patients. Also, healthcare providers must become informed and comfortable with using HHT applications instead of more traditional and costly approaches to case management. Medical schools must provide students with hands-on experience in managing patients through electronic telecommunication appli-cations in much the same way they prepare students to use hy-brid versions of this technology in both diagnostic and surgical applications. The transition to managing disease and promoting wellness using HHT applications requires paradigm shifts in healthcare delivery and education.

Since a small percentage of computer-equipped households have access to network services, the telephone remains the most likely alternative link because it can provide similar communi-cation functions. Approximately 93% of American households have at least one telephone. Public telephone networks have the most extensive coverage. With modifications in equipment, data, images, and slow-speed video can be transmitted over home telephone lines. Chapter Four provides more details on dis-parate, integrated HHT applications, including a review of five point-of-care systems.

The telephone should be used to its fullest capacity to meet healthcare needs until a better standard integrated healthcare information system is established (which, according to experts, may realistically take at least another decade).

DIGITIZING HEALTHCARE

By 1986, the potential of the telephone was expanded by Integrated Services Digital Network (ISDN) technology, which has become a widely used method of digital transmission using regular telephone lines and the public switched telephone network. ISDN systems now offer high-speed data, sound, graphics, and low-quality video at a small fraction of the cost of the super-cable TV systems. Cost is the Achilles' heel of implementing a system with information on demand and distance learning. Without a mass market, ISDN may remain too costly for the vast majority of healthcare providers and consumers until the demand for such services is sufficient to create a level of use that will demonstrate cost benefits. The recent use of Asymmetric Digital Subscriber Line (ADSL) modems, which are even faster than ISDN, enables simultaneous phone and Internet connection while keeping voice and data communications separate. The cable television industry is also making the transition to providing digital connections to homes using cable modems. The competitive nature of the electronics industry should facilitate the development, application, and use of digital technology into the next century.

INTEGRATING TELECOMMUNICATIONS INTO HEALTHCARE

The term *telemedicine* originated in the academic community. Telemedicine consists of a range of technologies and clinical applications that integrate and transfer information from one location to another using electronic signals. The type of information transferred and the technology used empirically define telemedicine. The transfer of images in radiology (i.e., teleradiology) and pathology (i.e., telepathology) were among the first applications in the 1970s. Many people saw the potential of telemedicine to meet specialty care needs in underserved areas. Additional benefits include more efficient use of resources, community outreach, and attracting international use of America's healthcare services. Although the use of telemedicine in general has proven to be cost effective, early skeptics viewed it as an inappropriate use of limited healthcare funds.

By simply examining the costs of reducing patients' office, emergency room, and hospital visits, through the use of the ordinary telephone, the financial benefits are obvious and indisputable. The telephone alone has consistently proven to be effective in providing quality, cost-effective home health-care through a variety of applications.[5]

Initially, telemedicine provided the most benefit to those who had limited access to care or who required continuous access to information for proper medical management. A ubiquitous approach to telemedicine uses the ordinary telephone for consultation, information transfer, scheduling, and certain areas of patient management. In addition to providing diagnostic and therapeutic consultation using still and video images, telemedicine is becoming increasingly effective in providing medical education and case management documentation.

Most households have touch-tone telephones that provide immediate connection to automated services and centers staffed by healthcare professionals. The opportunities are there; however, the technology is complex and unformed. Digital telephone technology is likely to increase over the next few years, and it has the potential of dramatically reducing both human and financial costs. The goals are health enhancing, profitable, and accessible.

A standardized, lifelong, integrated electronic clinical record is today a reality that unfortunately is underutilized. Ultimately, technology will enable both initiation and updating from the patient's home. Patient histories will be assessed with the assistance of a nurse or physician assistant using an on-line telephone, prior to scheduling visits. A continuum of care beginning with the patient at home, utilizing a computer-telephone or computer, makes more sense than waiting for the patient to come to the physician's office with a complaint.

Patients given responsibility learn to appreciate the value of accurate data collection and symptom reporting. Using electronic management facilitates the transfer of data, avoids duplication, and provides real-time access to information and support. Searching relevant databases (e.g., knowledge resources and decision-support services) facilitates the role of patients as care partners. Also, they are able to scan the professional profiles of healthcare providers. In the near future, outcome data will be available to patients and their caregivers so that true informed consent can be achieved—a common goal in managed care. All of these things can be achieved by linking care providers and patients through HHT.

Broadband networks using primarily fiber-optic cable, which has the highest bandwidth transmission capability, will provide the capability for worldwide information distribution. In the meantime, the opportunity to serve the masses with ISDN technology is being suppressed by those who believe in the high expectations and potential of broadband networks. The benefits of this system unfortunately are limited to the few who can afford such services. Within five years, the public switched telephone network combined with ISDN could serve the daily healthcare needs of all who have touch-tone telephones. This could be done at a fraction of the cost required for broadband networks, which will require several years to be constructed.

The *le minitel,* or Teletal, which is used widely in France, had been conceived mainly as an electronic telephone directory, reducing the need for printed directories and directory-assistance operators. By 1986, use of Teletal had expanded to over 2,000 on-line services. Chapter Five focuses on the role of this new digital "smart" telephone in home healthcare.

Providing timely, multimedia information using the digital phone, in user-friendly modules, to patients and their caretakers at home, in the language of their choice, is an essential component of any solution to many healthcare problems that require continuity of care, access, and clinical support.

Only five years ago, making health information available across an open network was merely a fantasy. With the combination of the digital telephone and the establishment of Community Healthcare Information Networks (CHINs), linking physicians to physicians, physicians to hospitals, hospitals to other institutions, and all to payers, is now possible. This one-step function will be highly advantageous to healthcare administrators. These links should include the home setting and the work site. Patients need to be an integral part as well. Too often patients do not realize that they are a vital part of the healthcare team. To participate more fully in their care, patients and providers must have access to information. Such links must respond to the need for both health and cost benefits.

COSTS AND BENEFITS

A review of the history of telemedicine and its impact on clinical and public health objectives shows that greater continuity of care and immediate cost benefits were evident in those applications that made use of telecommunications to reduce visits (Figure 2–2). Reduced days of stay and emergency room visits included patients with coronary heart disease, diabetes, psychiatric disorders, cancer, and single births. Reduced hospital readmissions included all of the above patient groups except single births.

The management of common chronic illnesses through the use of HHT is starting to show positive results in patient-based programs on early intervention and prevention. HHT applications have proven to be highly effective in persuading elderly patients to receive influenza vaccinations, take their medications, and comply to prescribed therapeutic activities.[6]

Rising costs have become a major force in the shift from traditional treatments to disease and care management models, in which patients must play a much bigger role than ever before.

FIGURE 2–2

Cost Benefits of Video Home Visits

Use of video visits	Cases	Potential amount saved
Home Health Services (20% of 100,000)	20,000	$600,000 Annually[a]
To reduce days of hospital stay	260	$243,000[b]
To reduce emergency room visits	875	$64,085[c]
To reduce hospital readmissions	2,135	$248,610[c]
Total		**$1,155,695**

[a]Indicates the average direct variable cost of providing service.
[b]10% shorter stay.
[c]10% less.

Source: HELP Innovations, Inc.: *Potential Cost Savings*, Lawrence, KS, August 1997.

Furthermore, case management requires teamwork, information, and communication to facilitate provider-patient partnering. In many settings, success may depend on the ability to inform, educate and motivate healthcare consumers by use of the telephone.

Telephones, facsimile machines, and computer systems continue to be part of the solutions to common communication problems in healthcare. Nearly one quarter of the population of the United States resides in remote or underserved areas. Telemedicine has extensively and effectively reached this population by way of the standard telephone.

THE 1996 TELECOMMUNICATIONS ACT

The 1996 Telecommunications Act was an important first step toward meeting the communication needs of healthcare. The Act provides universal service support only to eligible rural healthcare providers that match the following criteria:

- Not-for-profit hospitals
- Post-secondary educational institutions providing healthcare instruction
- Local health departments and agencies
- Health centers that provide care to migrants
- Rural clinics
- Healthcare consortia consisting of one or more of the above

Certain types of visits to physicians' offices, emergency rooms, hospitals, and skilled nursing facilities will continue. On the other hand, many physician–patient interactions, especially those seeking and offering information, could be conducted far more accurately and efficiently at home. Unfortunately, there is no incentive among fee-for-service physicians to encourage expanded home care services. Since physicians are compensated for seeing patients in their offices or institutional settings, a paradigm shift without economic incentives is unrealistic. A financial support structure that will reward physicians for effectively using home care options is needed.

By increasing the use of digital technology, HHT has the potential to link physicians with patients at home, significantly expanding home healthcare, which is well worth exploring as part of any financial support plan. The financial and legal aspects alone appear to be impeding the process of building the "information superhighway."

Until the necessary battles are fought and resolutions are made, the Internet will continue to move the digital world slower than necessary due to the expanding demand for its use. The ultimate solution to this communication problem should be cost-effective, long-range, and capable of facilitating networking and partnering among communication leaders. Access to healthcare information at a reasonable cost will eventually accelerate the demand. As patients are increasingly required to play a more active role in disease prevention as well as disease management, access to information will become a mandate. While these preliminary issues are being resolved, other digital telecommunications technologies present another option recommended by international telecommunications organizations. This network concept provides users of telecommunications services with digital access to integrated voice, data, and video applications. Europe is far ahead of the United States in the movement to digitize communication networks.

It is fair to assume that the home telephone remains the backbone of communication technology that improves access to and coordination of clinical care. Many applications of the telephone to home healthcare have been used and found to be cost effective in addition to facilitating disease management as evidenced by the evaluation of patient outcomes. Around-the-clock telephone access to healthcare providers has proved to be a cost-effective way to clarify instructions, provide emergency consultations, and give emotional support. Fewer days spent in the hospital, fewer outpatient visits, and higher levels of patient satisfaction are consistently reported. Because of the lack of appropriate research, the balance of evidence is insufficient to determine the true cost benefits of telemedicine in many of the more sophisticated areas of application. Nevertheless, the telephone remains the universal instrument of telemedicine applications.

Knowledgeable consumers have more options, take more responsibility, and make better choices. The cost benefits of preventing just one case of hepatitis are staggering. An awareness of one's options, particularly risk factors, can promote the total physical, social, and mental well-being of all people, while at the same time reducing the costs of healthcare to the individual and society.

HHT PATHFINDING HINTS

Where does one go from here in making decisions about HHT? Through the use of various integrated applications, HHT should be able to serve the medical needs of patients, guide and track healthcare providers, transfer information, and recommend care. When making choices about developing or procuring HHT applications, the following hints on the kinds of features to look for should prove helpful.[7]

Risk Stratification

Risk stratification requires the generation of a daily list of each patient's problems, medications, allergies, diagnostic tests, and home visits. Ultimately, the stratification of individual and family risk factors should be included.

Clinical Guidelines Implementation

Clinical guidelines implementation supports the use of clinical guidelines at the reference, reminder, and automated levels. The reference level includes all information in the patient's database, which is used routinely by healthcare providers. Prompts at the very moment of clinical decision-making about tests, medications, referrals, or therapies constitute the reminder level. The automated level includes capabilities related to clinical policy making, a critical part of establishing practices and protocols, and providing quality care. Also, on-line access to medical publications, decision-making models, cost-effectiveness information, and clinical policies should be considered important features to come in the future.

Care Coordination

Care coordination among all providers has been essential since the advent of managed care. Approaches that focus on utilization management are more appropriate than the gatekeeper model. All team members should have access to the same information, making the coordination of care more effective. For example, abnormal test results obtained from a homebound patient should automatically go to the appropriate clinical team member.

Patient Compliance

Patient compliance is one of the biggest concerns in home healthcare. HHT applications that ensure patient compliance with protocols are essential. Patient advisories, rewards, surveillance of certain medical screenings, clinical monitoring, patient access to information, support services, and patient itineraries are all part of the desirable features for patient compliance. Additional features worth consideration include electronically routed lab and radiology results, verifications, and clinical advice functions.

When selecting HHT applications, the strategy should be to determine what to keep, what to discard, and what to add. Applications involving disease or care management should be included. Such integration usually involves a process of procuring new technology, which starts by identifying and prioritizing needs in combination with what is affordable.

CONCLUSION

One of the biggest challenges of opening the door to digital technologies is the problems associated with their use in HTT. The opportunities to create solutions to old and new problems in home healthcare are endless. "Me too" solutions that maintain the status quo are more likely to be replaced by solutions that address cost benefits and provider satisfaction and truly make a difference. The role of the patient has drastically changed because of healthcare reform. Patients are now more important than ever in achieving optimal levels of health through home-based education and care. The magic has never been in the technology itself. It resides in those who lead the way in how best to use digital technology in the business of home healthcare.

REFERENCES

1. A History of the Telephone, prepared by Dawn M. Flammger, February, 1995, *tele2.html* at *www.geog.buffalo.edu*.
2. Ibid.
3. Nathan Fine: *Labor and Farmer Parties in the United States, 1828–1928,* p. 129, New York, 1938, Rand School of Social Science.
4. E. Andrew Balas, Farad J., Gilad J.K., et al.: Electronic Communication With Patients: Evaluation of Distance Medicine Technology, *JAMA* 278(no. 2), 1997, pp. 152–159.
5. Ibid.
6. HELP Innovations, Inc.: *Potential Cost Savings,* Lawrence, KS, August 1997.
7. Sue Auxter: Designing Information Systems for Disease Management: Moving from Disparate to Integrated Systems, *Clinical Laboratory News* 24(no. 4), 1998, pp. 1, 4–5.

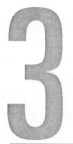

CHAPTER

The Business of Home Healthcare

INTRODUCTION AND PURPOSES

Successfully competing in the home healthcare industry takes effective leadership, management, knowledge of the industry, and the ability to respond quickly to new challenges. As a business, home healthcare represents a growing sector of the larger healthcare industry, and one of increasing importance. With significant government regulation and intervention, change has become the new watchword for those leading their companies. Given the concerted efforts to control spending, professionals must be creative about how they provide high-quality services while still remaining economically viable.

The purpose of this chapter is to describe the nature of the home healthcare business to frame the roles and opportunities for greater use of telecommunications later in this book. More specifically, the goals of this chapter are to:

- Acquaint you with several of the characteristics and reference points effective managers utilize to run their businesses

- Provide an overview of the healthcare delivery system, including the movement of the industry to managed care
- Characterize the structure of the home healthcare industry
- Identify the major challenges facing the industry
- Introduce the role that telecommunications can play in responding to the industry's challenges

HOMECARE AS A BUSINESS

Successfully running a business in home healthcare depends on some generic planning, management and leadership skills, combined with a passion for performance, and the ability to navigate the turbulent tides that seem to continually rock the industry. The pressures are mounting daily, and it seems that there is more and more uncertainty about what to do.

At one level, the business of home healthcare is like any other: one must offer a service that is needed by your customers, at a quality level they expect, and at a price that covers costs and results in some profit. Doing all of these things requires a high degree of organization and planning as well as an ability to know whether one is on track.

Owners and senior managers are the driving forces in running a successful home healthcare business. As leaders, they focus on objectives and make decisions that set a course of action for the agency's operations. They plan and set policies that anticipate future needs and find alternative courses of action. They organize and staff their organizations with the proper people, resources, tools, technologies, and workflow plans to get the work done on schedule. Furthermore, they direct activity and measure performance over time to ensure that objectives are being met.

These functions are not unique to the home healthcare industry but instead serve as a baseline of attributes for all successful managers. However, when managers are placed in the context of the home healthcare industry, it is interesting to see how they do when things become more complicated.

Many characteristics of an industry or an organization are beyond the influence and control of a manager yet are critical to the job he or she must perform in the business world. The ability to recognize these factors often has a sizable impact on a manager's ability to respond in a timely way. Some of the complicating forces for managers to be aware of include:

Change and Resistance to Change

The manager's professional role is changing and yet is resistant to change. No two days are the same, and it is often hard to predict what crisis is coming next. Maintaining a routine can be difficult because circumstances often change. Many employees, however, often resist change because it causes uncertainty. Others seem to want change because it represents something different from the current (i.e., unsatisfying) routine. It is up to the manager, owner, or leader to develop processes to manage change and use it for the benefit of the agency.

Knowns and Unknowns

Managers face a world of the known and unknown factors. Because the manager must anticipate the future, it is almost certain that a great deal of what he or she has to do focuses on dealing with the unknown. It is hard to know whether one decision is better than another. Likewise, it is hard for managers to know everything they should about the people around them or what the government will do next to affect reimbursement.

Controllable and Uncontrollable Factors

Managers can have a direct impact on factors that can be controlled, and these factors can be positively linked to performance. However, the number of factors that cannot be controlled seems to be constantly increasing, making final outcomes less predictable. Managers have to adapt to forces they cannot influence and still make the best of the situation, particularly in a turbulent external environment such as home healthcare.

Opportunities and Risks

Sizing up and seizing opportunities using evidence and experience is an attribute to be treasured in executives. Innovative, effective managers are willing to take calculated risks to move their company forward and stay ahead of the competition. Similarly, recognizing which risks are not worth taking is another attribute that distinguishes effective leaders from those who are just average.

Another important concept for home healthcare managers to recognize is the life cycle of a business. Simply put, organizations have three major stages in their life cycle: a start-up stage, an operating stage, and a slow-down or "start-again" stage. Once a business gets started, it tends to grow. The second stage is the period when operations stabilize by making adjustments and surviving in a very competitive situation. The third stage has three possibilities. First, an organization that has been unable to adjust will move toward a slow death or bankruptcy, resulting in the termination of its existence. Or it may become innovative, with new ideas and new approaches to its problems. Finally, it may merge with other firms to start another growth cycle.

A knowledge of a company's position in the life cycle may help a manager in making decisions that are specific to the business. It can guide the selection of the type of employee (for example, people who do not like change generally do not like to be associated with start-up companies), the degree of risk that should be taken to meet the competition, or the mix of business to be pursued. Depending on the maturity of the company, its capital resources, and its overall ability to change, companies will react differently to the uncertain, uncontrollable nature of the external environment, and they will prosper or flounder as a result.

The final characteristic of an effective home healthcare manager is having a high degree of knowledge about the industry. That means understanding the dynamics and forces that impinge on the risk–reward matrix, an ability to spot trends, staying alert to the subtleties of client needs and demands, and the ability to evaluate the economic climate and structural changes in the industry. Effective managers must not only be able to react to these forces, but also must anticipate them and develop plans to forge a competitive position.

An intimate knowledge of the industry also guides decisions about the best business strategies to pursue. How far can one go with a telemedicine program and where can it be implemented? What are the barriers to entry for a better-funded competitor who takes aim on one's client base? Is the company too dependent on a limited number of client services? What will happen when the reimbursement scheme changes? These questions and many others must be assessed and answered in the context of the industry as a whole, the local economy, and the structure of the delivery system in the region served.

In thinking further about what it takes to run a successful home healthcare company, the authors consulted with one of the country's outstanding business leaders, Thomas Tucker, President of Medline Homecare, Inc., and asked him what it is that makes a difference in the success of a company. Medline is a major manufacturer and distributor of homecare supplies, and as such, it is in close contact with all of the entities in the industry.

After considering the current landscape, Tucker defined the following distinguishing characteristics of successful companies:

- The ability to react quickly to the industry-wide challenges regarding reimbursements, shifting markets (into managed care), greater regulation, etc.
- The ability to make necessary changes, to re-engineer their processes (without fear or trepidation), and to develop a fresh approach to service delivery
- The ability to reduce overhead and manage costs while maintaining quality service levels
- The necessity of implementing data systems that enable proactive, customer-oriented decision-making

Tucker also had useful advice for other sectors of the industry beyond the agency level. He urged suppliers to help their customers control costs, and thus serve their patients better. Where opportunities exist, suppliers should seek out and sell into new markets (e.g., mail-order), and generally help improve overall management of costs by using data and information management resources to improve the delivery of goods. They should create better interface systems between themselves and their customers, manage the information support process, and take advantage of the new electronic capacities that are now readily available. The telephone, Internet telephones, telemedicine/telehealth technologies, and electronic ordering are among the many innovations that provide the tools to make job response faster and more efficient.

Furthermore, Tucker suggested that durable medical equipment (DME) providers should concentrate on integrating provider and patient information and finding ways to empower patients to participate in the care process. Much of this can be accomplished by enabling patients to enter data from their homes using simple access devices.

Tucker's advice rings true in an era of steep competition, and it comes from a successful professional who has been "in the trenches" for years.

The previous discussion provides a brief look at some of the components necessary for building a successful home healthcare business, including the pivotal role of the owner or manager. The following text provides an examination of the specifics of the overall industry and an identification of the issues that are creating the biggest challenges to successful operation.

OVERVIEW OF THE HEALTHCARE DELIVERY SYSTEM

The U.S. healthcare delivery system is massive, fragmented, and fragile. Its key players (i.e., healthcare providers, patients, and payers) are diverse and often have conflicting needs. Hospitals consume over one third of the healthcare budget, but most are struggling to maintain financial viability in the wake of industry changes. Tens of thousands of ambulatory care facilities have arisen to compete with hospitals for patient dollars. These facilities, including physicians' offices, hospital-based outpatient clinics and emergency rooms, ambulatory care centers, free-standing outpatient surgical centers and specialized clinics, often provide more cost-efficient care and serve as an entry point to more complex care. In addition, thousands of nursing homes and homecare agencies provide long-term care services to the growing elderly population.

The financing of healthcare is split among the government, employers, and individuals. There are a number of intermediaries, such as insurance companies, but fundamentally, all of the dollars in the system essentially come from these three sources. Creating an awareness among these groups about the way care is delivered and ensuring cost-efficient operation provide an ongoing benchmark for providers and patients.

The healthcare system has been strained to the breaking point because of the nation's need to improve access to quality care, and to reduce total costs. The growing size and complexity of the industry has had a dramatic effect on the growth of resource consumption. Expenditure growth will continue as the population ages and as new technologies and drugs prolong patients' lives and better control patient outcomes. In addition, patients often have unrealistic expectations for the "cure." Until outcomes are routinely and clearly reported and patient expectations can be aligned with medical realities, expenditures will continue to increase.

Employers are a principal contributor to healthcare spending in the U.S., and they are under increasing pressure from the government to assume a larger portion of this obligation. Employers have a vested interest in ensuring the long-term health of their work force, but these benefits are expensive. Furthermore, there is a limit to the extent employees are willing to share this burden—medical benefits are often a principal bargaining point in labor negotiations. Both individuals and businesses are increasingly turning back to the government to demand policies that will resolve this dilemma.

The federal and state governments have attempted to respond to the three important, but often conflicting, demands in healthcare—cost, quality, and access—in various ways. Major reform bills have been introduced, new regulations have been implemented, and the industry itself has responded with structural changes. The movement toward managed care, the emergence of integrated delivery networks, the development of specialized niche providers, including home healthcare, and the impact of the government seem to be the main impetus in efforts to reconcile the demands of cost, quality, and access.

THE MOVEMENT TOWARD MANAGED CARE

Healthcare expenditures in the U.S. for 1997 were estimated to be $1.09 trillion.[1] Growth has slowed over the last few years, and expenditures are expected to increase by less than 6% per year over the next decade, according to the Congressional Budget Office. The major factor driving the moderation in cost growth has been the move toward managed care as a payment mechanism.

More and more employees are moving into managed care, and this shift has led to price competition in the marketplace. As a result, employers' healthcare plan costs were nearly stable in 1997.

A survey by Mercer/Foster Higgins revealed that group healthcare costs for active and retired employees were $3,924 per employee in 1997.[2] For larger employers (i.e., those with over 500 employees), the average cost was $4,369 per employee. The average cost for HMO membership was significantly less, at around $3,165 per active employee per year.[3]

However, this relatively calm period in price escalation may be ending. Large numbers of individuals have already moved into managed care plans, and the cost savings relative to indemnity programs have been realized. In addition, many HMOs that have held their rates artificially low to win market share are now raising rates to improve their financial results.

Another factor affecting the market is the movement of retirees into managed care plans. In 1997 the percentage of early retirees with employer-provided coverage nearly doubled from the previous year (from 15% to 26%).[4] Medicare-eligible retirees enrolled in managed care plans represented 25% of those individuals with employer-provided coverage (up from 17% in 1996).[5] The cost savings from these shifts could be dramatic, both for the employer and the retiree.

Managed care has had and will continue to have profound effects on the economic structure of the industry and perceptions about the quality of care rendered to patients. Its impact on home healthcare is dramatic because it will increasingly affect those who are the biggest users of homecare services. Furthermore, these changes will continue to drive more people into home healthcare and lead to more growth in the industry.

HOME HEALTHCARE IN THE UNITED STATES

The concern over accelerating costs has created a new imperative: patient care must be provided in the most cost-effective environment, consistent with quality standards. This evolution, along with the growth of the elderly population in the U.S., makes home healthcare an attractive alternative to institutional forms of care.

   With the aging population comes an increase in healthcare concerns and costs. To control rising costs, payers are demanding shorter hospital stays; consequently, patients are being sent home earlier. Surgeries once considered to be quite serious, such as hysterectomies, are now done on an outpatient basis. Even patients undergoing multiple heart bypass surgeries are being sent home in a matter of days. Mothers are being sent home as early as eight hours after giving birth.

   Because patients are often ill prepared for the days following surgery or childbirth, healthcare providers and insurance companies are seeking innovative ways to meet expectations for accessible, affordable, and high-quality healthcare. Home healthcare offers attractive options for consumers, insurers, and hospitals alike.

   Many patients eagerly go home from the hospital thinking they can manage by themselves. At home they are often faced with a new set of issues that make the hospital-to-home transition overwhelming. Patients may have thought they understood the doctors' orders, such as how and when to take the medication, or thought they would be able to easily maneuver stairs or cook for themselves. However, things may be "different" once they go home. This situation is common.

   In response to these challenges, a number of healthcare services are now available at home . . . and not just for elderly patients. Home healthcare agencies, however, are not all alike. A few provide the full range of services, but some agencies provide only medical equipment, such as walkers or wheelchairs, while others focus on high-tech services, such as in-home chemotherapy, hydration, or tube feedings. Still others simply provide companionship and basic services, such as shopping, meal preparation, and bathing. Registered nurses conduct post-natal follow-up visits for new mothers and babies. High-tech services, such as antibiotic intravenous therapy, allow patients to receive treatment conveniently, privately, and affordably. Physical and occupational therapists can work with patients in their own environments to help them get around and accomplish daily tasks.

   Receiving care in the home is not only affordable but also allows for quality, personalized attention and the comfort of knowing that the patient's condition is monitored daily. Home healthcare focuses on getting the individual back to good health so he or she can enjoy a life that is as fulfilling and independent as possible—all in the privacy, comfort, and convenience of familiar surroundings.

Home healthcare in the United States continues to be a diverse and rapidly growing service industry. There are nearly 15,000 providers delivering services to over 7 million people, who require help because of acute illnesses, chronic health conditions, permanent disabilities, or terminal illnesses. Annual expenditures for home healthcare were in excess of $42 billion in 1997.[6]

While $42 billion is certainly a lot of money, it represents only about 4% of the total spending on personal healthcare in the U.S. What captures people's attention, however, is the projected growth of home healthcare to 10% of total spending over the next decade. This dramatic growth will result from all the previously stated reasons why the home is an excellent site for care, as well as the inherent cost efficiencies associated with it.

The tone from government analysts suggests some alarm about the rate of growth for home healthcare. However, this growth may be appropriate, not only for patients, but for the economy as well. Perhaps home healthcare should represent an even greater percentage of the total if it is truly more efficient and able to provide quality care, while other sectors of the healthcare industry (like hospitals) should reduce their overall expenditures.

Fully one half of the homecare providers are Medicare-certified home healthcare agencies according to the HCFA.[7] Hospital-based and freestanding proprietary agencies have grown faster than any other type of certified agency, and they now represent about 75% of the total number of agencies. Medicare is the largest single payer of home healthcare services, accounting for nearly one half of the total expenditures. Other public funding sources for home healthcare include Medicaid, the Older Americans Act, Title XX Social Services Block Grants, the Veterans' Administration, and the Civilian Health and Medical Program of the Uniformed Services (CHAMPUS). Private insurance comprised only a small portion of home healthcare payments. Table 3–1 shows the sources of payment for home healthcare in 1995.

TABLE 3–1

Sources of Payment for Home Healthcare (1996)

Source of Payment	Percentage of Total Expenditures
Medicare	65.2
Medicaid	9.6
Private insurance and self-pay	13.6
Other/unknown	11.6

Source: Agency for Health Care Policy and Research, Center for Cost and Financing Studies, *National Medical Expenditure Survey Data (Aligned to National Health Accounts Data),* Rockville, MD, March 1997, AHCPR.

Home healthcare is a very efficient way to provide medical services, and this efficiency is a major reason for its projected growth. Table 3–2 shows the average cost per visit.

The increase in the number of Medicare beneficiaries is also propelling growth in home healthcare services. In 1997, HCFA estimated that 38.6 million aged and disabled people were enrolled in the Medicare program.[8] About 10% of these enrollees received home healthcare services that year—twice the number from 1990. Table 3–3 shows the growth in Medicare home healthcare benefits.

TABLE 3–2

Average Cost Per Home Healthcare Visit (1987 and 1997)

	1987	1997[a]
Nurse	$62	$98
Therapist	$57	$90
Home healthcare aide	$34	$54
Homemaker	$33	$52
Other[b]	$56	$89
Average	**$48**	**$77**

[a]Updated by the average annual rate of increase of Medicare per-visit charges, which was 4.7% between 1987 and 1995 (HCFA, Office of Information Services).

[b]Includes social workers and other professionals.

Source: Altman, B., Walden, D.: *Home Health Care: Use, Expenditures and Sources of Payment,* National Medical Expenditure Survey Research Findings 15, Pub. No. 93-0040, Rockville, MD, 1993, AHCPR.

TABLE 3–3

Medicare Home Healthcare Outlays, Clients, and Visits (1990–1997)

Year	Outlays (in Millions of Dollars)	Clients (in 1000s)	Visits (in 1000s)
1990	3,860	1,940	69,532
1991	5,566	2,223	99,183
1992	7,859	2,523	134,877
1993	10,263	2,868	169,142
1994	13,347	3,175	220,693
1995	16,223	3,570	266,438
1996	18,060	3,735	285,826
1997	20,465	3,910	306,116

Source: HCFA, Office of the Actuary and Bureau of Data Management and Strategy. *1997 Report,* Washington, D.C., 1997, Government Printing Office. Note: The data from 1990 to 1997 was updated February 10, 1997 for Medicare Trustees Report.

Most of the growth in spending has occurred as a result of the increase in the number of visits (from 70 million in 1990 to 306 million in 1997).[9] Growth in Medicare home healthcare benefits can be attributed to specific legislative expansions of the benefits and to a number of socio-demographic trends, which have fostered growth in the program from the beginning and will no doubt continue to do so for many years to come. With reimbursement based on visits as the primary incentive, it is not surprising that the number of visits has grown so dramatically. Businesses quickly learn to align their operations with the incentives available to them.

There are six types of visits that are covered by Medicare: skilled nursing, physical therapy, occupational therapy, speech therapy, medical social services, and home healthcare aides. The Balanced Budget Act of 1997 introduced new limits designed to reduce growth in Medicare expenditures for home healthcare, and these new regulations will have a sizeable impact on the industry. These changes will be discussed later in this chapter.

WHO ARE HOME HEALTHCARE PATIENTS?

Estimates indicate that as many as 9 to 11 million Americans need home healthcare services.[10] Most will receive services from so-called informal caregivers, including family members, friends, or others who provide services on an unpaid basis.

Projections from a National Association for Medical Equipment Services (NAMES) study suggest that 7.4 million individuals received home healthcare services in 1997.[11] Of these recipients, nearly one half were over the age of 65, and the amount of care they received tended to increase with age. About 40% of the recipients had functional limitations in one or more activities of daily living. Age and functional disability are likely predictors of the need for home healthcare services.

The leading reasons for people receiving home healthcare services were conditions related to diseases of the circulatory system (30%) and heart disease, including congestive heart failure (20%). The remainder were predominately from stroke, diabetes, and hypertension victims.[12]

WHO ARE THE CAREGIVERS?

Both informal and formal caregivers are important to the system of rendering care at home.[13] Estimates indicate that almost three quarters of elderly persons with severe disabilities receiving home healthcare services in 1989 relied solely on family members or other unpaid help.[14] Eight of 10 informal caregivers provide unpaid assistance for an average of 4 hours per day, 7 days per week. Three quarters of informal caregivers are female, and nearly one third are older than 65.[15]

A 1996 telephone survey estimated that there were 22 million U.S. households with at least one member who provided some level of unpaid assistance to a spouse, relative, or other person older than age 50.[16] These services are almost without exception provided by individuals with little training, technological support, or access to important information.

Formal caregivers include professionals and paraprofessionals who provide home healthcare and personal care services and are compensated for the services they provide. The Bureau of Labor Statistics (BLS) and HCFA provide data on these employees. However, agency definitions and methods of counting are different. BLS provides an occupational classification for "home healthcare services" that excludes hospital-based and public agency workers. Its method of counting is "the number of employees." HCFA limits its statistics to employees of Medicare-certified home healthcare agencies. Furthermore, its survey presents data on full-time equivalents (FTEs).

BLS estimated that more than 500,000 people were employed in home healthcare agencies in 1994, with the exclusions described above (Table 3–4). HCFA counted 404,959 FTEs employed in Medicare-certified agencies at the end of 1996. Using either method, the largest numbers of employees are home healthcare aides and RNs.

Table 3–5 shows the yearly employment numbers for home healthcare services for 1991–1996 based on BLS monthly statistics. During the period 1991–1996, home healthcare employment grew from 344,000 employees to 669,000 employees—a 14% annual rate of growth.

TABLE 3–4

Number of Home Healthcare Employees (1994)[1] and Medicare-Certified Agency FTEs (1996)[2]

Type of Employee	Number of Home Healthcare Employees	Number of FTEs
Registered nurses	112,217	144,390
Licensed practical nurses	39,774	32,733
Physical therapists	9,378	13,651
Home healthcare aides	242,291	136,495
Occupational therapists	3,626	3,569
Speech pathologists	2,758	2,096
Social workers	7,508	7,489
Other	137,848	64,536
Totals	**555,400**	**404,959**

Sources: [1]U.S. Department of Labor, Bureau of Labor Statistics: *National Industry-Occupation Employment Matrix (1994)*, Washington, D.C., 1996. (Excludes hospital-based and public agencies.); [2]Unpublished data on FTEs in Medicare-certified home healthcare agencies as of December 1996. From the HCFA Center for Information Systems, Health Standards and Quality Bureau.

T A B L E   3–5

Home Healthcare Services Total Employment (1991–1996)

Year	Total Number of Employees
1991	344,000
1992	398,000
1993	469,000
1994	555,000
1995	610,000
1996	669,000

Note: Excludes hospital-based and public home healthcare agency employees.

Sources: HCFA: *Health Care Financing Review,* Summer 1996; U.S. Department of Labor, Employment and Earnings: *Establishment Data, 1991–1995,* U.S. Department of Labor, Bureau of Labor Statistics: *Establishment Data,* 1996, Washington, D.C.

Clearly, home healthcare is among the fastest growing segments of the health services industry. Employment has almost doubled since 1991. In comparison, hospital employment increased by just 10%, and total healthcare industry employment has increased by only 31%.[17]

Because reimbursements are so closely tied to the number of visits made to the home, it is interesting to note that several studies about nursing productivity indicate that nurses visit an average of 5 homes per day. Nurses who specialize in pediatric care average 2.4 visits per day.[18]

One way to retain a competitive position in the industry is to increase the productivity of the professional staff by providing them with the means to see more patients when necessary, while developing ways for data and information to come out of the home without a visit. Telecommunications play an important role here, and this subject will be discussed further in this chapter.

However, home healthcare is already a very efficient way to deliver care. Table 3–6 compares the average Medicare charges on a per-day basis for hospitals and skilled nursing facilities (SNFs) to the average Medicare charge for home visits.

Cost-effectiveness, however, is not the only rationale for home healthcare. In fact, the best argument for home healthcare is that it is a humane and compassionate way to deliver

TABLE 3–6

Comparison of Hospital, Skilled Nursing Facility, and Home Health Medicare Charges (1994–1996)

Charges per Day	1994[a]	1995[a]	1996[b]
Hospital[b]	$1,754	$1,910	$1,965
Skilled nursing facility[b]	356	402	414
Home health [c]	83	84	86

Sources: [a]Data are from Social Security Bulletin, Annual Statistical Supplement, 1994 and 1995; [b]Estimates for 1996 based on consumer price index for urban consumers from *The Economic and Budget Outlook*, Congressional Budget Office, January 1997; [c]HCFA, Office of Information Services.

healthcare and supportive services. Home healthcare reinforces and supplements the care provided by family members and friends and maintains the recipient's dignity and independence, which are too often lost—even in the best institutions. Furthermore, home healthcare allows patients to take an active role in their own care, becoming members of the multidisciplinary healthcare team.[19]

INDUSTRY CHALLENGES

Home healthcare is a rapidly growing part of the healthcare industry, and its values and cost efficiencies suggest that it will continue to grow for some time. However, there are some significant challenges that leaders must respond to because of the economic and service delivery impacts they create. The effective use of telecommunications can help improve the response to these challenges by home healthcare professionals.

Three issues currently dominate the home healthcare industry: reimbursement policies, planning in the face of uncertainty, and marketing and operations strategies.

Reimbursement Policies

Shrinking reimbursements are the most economically threatening issue for the home healthcare industry. Having to receive less money while providing the same services places enormous stress on every part of the system and requires unusually strong action to ensure business viability.

The Interim Payment System (IPS) raises concerns for both beneficiaries and providers of home healthcare services. This system will be in effect for fiscal years 1998 and 1999, after which it will be replaced by the Prospective Payment System (PPS). The National Association for Home Care (NAHC) calls the IPS the "most sweeping change in the way home health agencies have been reimbursed that have occurred since the program's inception in 1965."[20] Under the IPS, agencies are paid the lowest of their actual allowable costs, new reduced cost limits, or new per beneficiary limits.

The IPS requires that agencies hold down their costs without regard to past efficiency or current patient mix. It places tight limits on per beneficiary payments and can force agencies to reduce the frequency of visits or the number of staff members treating the most chronically ill patients. It may punish agencies in rural or other areas that are unable to balance high-cost patients with low-end users in order to remain under the payment limits. Agencies that cannot make cost reductions in the short term will likely experience financial losses and potentially close.

The Lewin Group Report raised concerns about the impact of the IPS on the access to care, shifting care to less appropriate settings, the lack of alternative financing sources, increases in beneficiary out-of-pocket payments, and the overall quality of care.[21] Most home healthcare agencies will need to reduce the cost per visit and cost per patient. Since nearly 78% of agencies' costs are labor related, these reductions in the payment ceilings could mean that agencies will have to reduce personnel, and for those who remain, may not be able to increase employee wages/fringe benefits to keep pace with cost of living increases, thereby reducing their attractiveness to current and potential employees. There are also pressures to reduce the number of services provided, which could have a more direct impact on home healthcare patients.

The legitimate concerns about the impact of the IPS must be weighed against the need for agencies to change and employ new techniques and technologies to survive and remain viable. The Lewin Report goes on to suggest that the following strategies are available to agencies:[22]

- Where medically appropriate, home healthcare agencies could reduce the number of visits provided to patients by targeting high-use patients for reductions.
- Home healthcare agencies could reduce their average number of visits and cost per user without rationing care by increasing the number of persons served, focusing on individuals who require less than the average numbers of visits. However, any additional patients would still be required to meet the Medicare coverage guidelines, so the pool of potential new home healthcare users may be limited.
- Home healthcare agencies could reduce their average number of visits and costs per patient by serving fewer high-use/high-cost patients. As a result, these patients may have difficulty accessing home healthcare services which increases the pressure on other settings, such as nursing homes and hospitals, or other payers such as state Medicaid programs.
- Home healthcare agencies could use several substitution strategies to reduce the average cost per beneficiary. These strategies include: reducing more expensive visits in favor of lower-cost visits where appropriate (e.g., substituting licensed practical nurses for registered nurses and therapy assistants for therapists); combining services within one visit when possible; and using telephone follow-up.
- Home healthcare agencies could establish care protocols and frequent status reviews in an effort to limit the possibility of providing excessive numbers of visits.

Home healthcare agencies will have to adopt one or more of these strategies to remain economically viable in the short term. Current processes will have to be re-engineered to conform to the constraints of the IPS (and eventually the PPS). Scrutinizing cost structures, providing more effective utilization management, changing personnel deployment, and effectively using telecommunications all become part of the re-engineering process. Good leadership at the agency level is essential.

Planning During Times of Uncertainty

Everyone agrees that planning is a fundamental management practice and is directly tied to the success of the business. Setting realistic goals, understanding the market forces, determining the most effective ways to get the job done, and executing a sound game plan are pivotal to on-going success. What makes the planning task so difficult is when there is so much uncertainty.

Uncertainty is bred, of course, by the industry's dependence on the government at a time when the government is changing the rules. Just as the IPS has created an urgency for change, the PPS, beginning in late 1999, will add another dimension of complexity.

The PPS is expected to be based on a per-episode payment adjusted for case mix. A per-episode PPS would require that agencies monitor the costs of care and the number of visits provided to beneficiaries, which is similar to the per-visit and per-beneficiary limits. However, payments would be adjusted to account for an agency's level of severity of clients served.

Regardless of what the final PPS regulations look like, the Balanced Budget Amendment of 1997 still requires that payment rates (both per-visit and per-beneficiary) be reduced by 15%. Agencies must immediately initiate steps to plan for these reductions and implement appropriate strategies to meet the new requirements.

Agencies must carefully define their markets and understand their client base (i.e., who they can serve and how well). They must make tough decisions about costs, seek aggressive ways to reduce these costs, and use their data, when it is available, to guide decisions, rather than basing significant business judgments on hunches.

Government efforts to reduce fraud and abuse add another element of uncertainty. Beginning with Operation Restore Trust (ORT), followed by the Wedge Project, and continuing with a variety of regulator-led fraud-busting strategies, agencies are under a great deal of pressure to demonstrate compliance.

Rooting out fraud and abuse is desirable, and certainly, these efforts are pursuing a laudable goal. Most industry veterans would agree that there have been instances of fraud and abuse, and these should be quickly eliminated. At the same time, most see the initiative as a way to create a political rationale to reduce expenditures and tighten up the documentation and management controls necessary for the industry to serve more people with less money.

The risk that comes with a heavy-handed approach, however, is that the public can become leery and develop a negative view of home healthcare. This could drive many individuals to seek hospital-based services again, which are far more expensive and are often not the medically appropriate level of care.

The implications of these antifraud activities are that agencies must find the financial resources and operational will to implement and maintain functional compliance or ethics programs within the constraints of the reimbursement limitations faced by the industry. Agencies that currently do so should benefit from training and employee communications modules that are central to functional programs. Well-designed training programs that provide employees with the tools to adjust to the IPS, the PPS, and tightened government oversight and which simultaneously spur innovation and creativity in program delivery are the precursors to successful agency operation.

Marketing Strategies

Shrinking reimbursements and greater market uncertainty have a great effect on the marketing and operation of home healthcare agencies. There are at least four impacts that need to be addressed.

Changes in Competitive Structure

The first of these effects that changes will occur in the competitive structure of the industry. There will also be changes in the agency incentives for the type of patients agencies would prefer to serve, and as a result, disruptions will occur in the established patterns of referrals. (Hospital discharge planners refer many home healthcare patients to an agency.) Each agency in a market tries to establish a particular niche in the market (e.g., high-tech care or care requiring home healthcare aides), and discharge planners and physicians will generally base referral patterns on the established strengths of agencies.

The growing trend toward hospitals referring their patients into their own home healthcare agencies creates alarm in many sectors of the industry. The Homecare Association of America (HCAA) called this matter the most critical issue facing independent agency owners.[23]

The HCAA position on patient choice is that patients should be allowed, without coercion or manipulation from hospital discharge staff, the freedom to choose his or her post-acute care provider, and that choice must be honored by the hospital and enforced by HCFA.[24] Independent agencies want a level playing field to compete for patients. At the same time, vertical integration by hospitals represents their competitive response to declining bed-days and the broader industry changes in the way care is administered and reimbursed.

Many agencies will attempt to move to higher levels of patient acuity to survive. Lower-level activities, while still important, will be handled more efficiently through emerging techniques that are less labor intensive. For example, the use of mail-order supplies, pharmaceuticals, and equipment allows for consolidation of current companies and the emergence of new ones that can specialize in these functions.

It will take time for the agencies, physicians, and the hospital discharge planners to reconfigure referral patterns in response to the new system. In addition, the per-beneficiary limits may vary substantially within the same market, encouraging agencies with higher per-beneficiary limits to market their services based on an ability to provide more services than competitors. This may put the agencies with a low cost per patient ratio in the base year at a competitive disadvantage.

Meeting competitive challenges ultimately depends on the quality of service provided, the cost of those services, and the positioning (e.g., reputation, track-record, value-added features, and location) of the organization among its competitors. Finding competitive advantages is crucial in every industry and every business. Later in the book, the authors propose that the effective use of telecommunications is one compelling way for an agency to achieve its competitive advantage in its market.

New Data Requirements

The second impact involves new data requirements. Because the Balanced Budget Act requires that agencies submit additional information for the development of a reliable case mix system, and because agencies must have a better understanding of their cost/profit structure, agencies must implement systems that electronically collect, sort, and analyze the appropriate data. The ability to systematically collect assessment and outcome data is required to achieve the positioning in the marketplace that is necessary from a marketing and operations perspective.

More Responsive Data Systems

The third impact is the need to develop more responsive data systems. For agencies to effectively manage care under the new payment system, they will need systems to track care provided to beneficiaries more closely. Agencies will also have a more immediate need for information in order to monitor the financial implications of the type and level of care provided. Agencies that have incorporated Outcomes and Assessment Information Set (OASIS) data collection into their system will be ahead of the game.

Similarly, response time is critical. Responses to patients, regulator inquiries, suppliers, and changing market conditions all demand a new sense of urgency and timeliness; only the nimble will survive. Again, the ability to act based on data will distinguish agencies from one another and increase the probability that their actions are correct. A strong data system is an investment that pays off many times over during turbulent times.

New Opportunities

The fourth impact of the changes in the industry is to realize that there are new opportunities as a result of these changes.

Those providers who are willing to change, can move quickly, and are willing to embrace innovation are going to survive. This means using effective data systems to collect and respond to the demands of patients, payers, and families and using telecommunications to reduce costs, when appropriate (particularly telecommunications devices that can be accessed from the home so that patients can participate in their own care).

For DME providers, developing a sales and marketing strategy that positions them to identify, target, and secure managed Medicare accounts is likely to be to their benefit. By carefully assessing the local market and presenting themselves as providing value-added services, at-risk contractors can offer ways to keep elderly patients healthier while reducing costs. For example, programs such as member satisfaction, case management, provider education, senior services, wellness exams, outcome measures, and disease management can be powerful selling tools for DME providers competing for managed Medicare contracts.

The overriding lessons to be learned are that the new home healthcare environment calls for agencies and DME providers to achieve a new level of data-based response, change, and innovation than ever before. Developing a passion for re-engineering the old ways of doing things, being willing to challenge assumptions that "it can't be done," and leading employees to provide exceptional care while achieving efficiencies will distinguish the successful players from those who find comfort in complaining.

THE ROLE OF TELECOMMUNICATIONS

The federal government and private insurers have applied numerous "band-aid" initiatives to slow the healthcare industry's skyrocketing costs. But no major national reforms have taken place, and there still has been little formal evaluation of the role telecommunications can play. Too much attention has been focused on the total medical bill instead of the root causes of the expenses and strategies that could improve the situation, such as health promotion, curtailing inappropriate treatments, and reducing administrative inefficiencies.

The healthcare industry has made astonishing gains in adopting advanced medical technology. It is far less progressive in its use of telecommunications and information technology to improve its traditional paper-intensive patient care, diagnostic, and clinical processes. The U.S. has not yet linked the telecommunications infrastructure to the healthcare infrastructure. To date, only local and regional pilots are in testing or operation. The results have been very promising, enough to suggest that a broader, more acceptable set of initiatives should be supported.

Healthcare providers are increasingly experimenting with expanded telecommunications applications that allow them to communicate with patients at home. These applications support the quality imperatives while also reducing costs. For example, telecommunications can reduce the amount of time a provider spends with patients for transmitting routine information, like normal test results. Telecommunications can also reduce visits to emergency rooms, doctor's offices, and hospitals because patients are directed to the appropriate level of care. Using telecommunications can allow for early intervention, offsetting more costly treatment after an episode requiring treatment. Furthermore, telecommunications can increase the productivity of home healthcare professionals, simplifying administrative duties, reducing the need for some visits, and providing better information in advance of a visit.

Many effective programs support one or more of the above benefits. Some programs supply patients with communications devices that allow them to signal for help in an emergency and, if necessary, receive treatment. Other companies supply miniaturized one-way communication, emergency response systems that patients can wear on their wrist or around their neck. When the patient falls, for example, he or she can press the button on the unit to trigger a call to the hospital, fire department, or emergency response center. Still others are using telemonitoring devices that allow patients to self-administer tests that normally require staff assistance to perform. Others use computerized terminals to direct the patient to the appropriate level of care based on his or her symptoms. More frequently, home healthcare professionals, such as nurses, carry units into the home after downloading the patient's information, then later, upload current status information to a central database.

PatientCare Technologies, Inc., based in Atlanta, is an innovator in using digital technology to support the home healthcare professional, as well as maintaining effective care management information and protocols. An excellent model of telehealth delivery that is appropriate to the specific needs of the patient is the ResourceLink system developed by HELP Innovations, Inc., of Lawrence, Kansas.

Innovations are cropping up quickly, presenting opportunities for companies that see the potential for gain while supporting patient care initiatives. New software systems permit integrated provider, patient, and supplier interaction. Development of information "infostructures," such as that developed by PatientCare Dynamics, Inc., of Mason, Ohio, provide a common standards-based platform at the physician's office that permits electronic linkage to the rest of the healthcare system. New generations of telephones, such as the CIDCO iPhone™, screen phones, and related Internet-based appliances, offer ease of use, inexpensive cost, and provide a platform that meets many of the needs of the industry from the patient's point of view. The advent of these devices is reason to be less sanguine about the role of expensive, high-maintenance devices that ultimately serve to distance the patient from being involved significantly in their own care.

As technologies improve, so does the potential for business opportunities for the innovators, cost reductions for the providers, and improved quality of care for the patients. The advent of remote consultations in both rural settings and the inner city, long-distance methodologies for training and continuing education, and opportunities for accessing the information and interactive resources of the Web from home all offer exciting new dimensions for the industry.

Although home healthcare has been buffeted by and continues to be a target of cost reductions, there are attractive opportunities for those who can effectively use the technologies to their own advantages—and to the advantage of their patients. The following chapters explore these opportunities in more detail and will provide a guide to the possibilities for the immediate future.

REFERENCES

1. Congressional Budget Office: *The Economic and Budget Outlook: Fiscal Years 1998–2002,* Washington, D.C., 1997, Congressional Budget Office.

2. Mercer/Foster Higgins: *National Survey of Employer-Sponsored Health Plans,* New York, 1988, Crain Communications.

3. Ibid.

4. Ibid.

5. Ibid.

6. Health Care Financing Administration, Center for Information Systems, Health Standards and Quality Bureau: *1997 Report,* Washington, D.C., 1997.

7. Health Care Financing Administration, Office of the Actuary: Unpublished estimates for the President's fiscal year 1998 budget. February 1997. Posted at *http://www.nahc.org/consumer/hestats.html.*

8. Health Care Financing Administration, Op. Cit.

9. Ibid.

10. U.S. Bipartisan Commission on Comprehensive Health Care: *The Pepper Commission Final Report: A Call for Action,* Op. Cit., pp. 101–104.

11. National Association for Medical Equipment Services: *National Medical Expenditure Survey, 1987,* New York, 1987.

12. Strahan, G.W.: *An Overview of Home Health and Hospice Care Patients: 1994 National Home and Hospice Care Survey,* National Center for Health Statistics, Washington, D.C., 1996.

13. U.S. Bipartisan Commission on Comprehensive Health Care: *The Pepper Commission Final Report: A Call for Action,* pp. 101–114, Washington, D.C., 1990, Government Printing Office.

14. Ibid.

15. Ibid.

16. National Alliance for Caregiving and the American Association for Retired Persons: *Family Caregiving in the U.S.: Findings From a National Survey,* Bethesda, MD, 1997, the Authors

17. HCFA, Officer of the Actuary, Op. Cit., p. 15.

18. Ibid., p. 16.

19. The Lewin Group: *The Lewin Report: Implications of the Medicare Home Health Interim Payment System of the 1997 Balanced Budget Act,* The National Association for Home Care, March 1997, Washington, D.C.

20. Ibid.

21. Ibid.

22. Ibid.

23. Homecare Association of America: *Position Paper Prepared for the Congress, 1996.* Posted at *http://hcaa-homecare.com/leg/cong1996.html.*

24. Ibid.

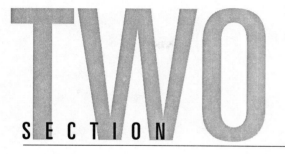

SECTION TWO

ADVANCES IN TECHNOLOGY

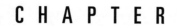

CHAPTER

Telecommunications in the Home

HOME HEALTH TELECOMMUNICATIONS

The delivery of healthcare is returning to the home. The application of telecommunications to home healthcare is a vast new frontier that has revolutionary implications. It has been many decades since local physicians made house calls, treating and keeping track of patients and families through routine home visits. House calls are like many other cultural practices, which often recycle. With the advent of managed care and high-tech/high-touch technology, home health telecommunications (HHT) is rapidly becoming a vital part of our healthcare system. It is fair to assume that electronic house calls are in everyone's future.

HHT encompasses the concepts of both telehealth and telemedicine. The use of computer and electronic information transfer technologies to promote health, prevent disease, educate consumers, access resources, and collect and manage data is referred to as telehealth. Telemedicine is the application of the same technologies to the delivery of medical care, including diagnosis, treatment, consultation, transfer of data, and interactive education and training. Because the transition to managed care relies on the global healthcare team approach, primary care physicians are now returning to both ambulatory and inpatient settings as care coordinators, partnering with their patients and families.

Those caregivers applying HHT technology are often referred to as home teleproviders, whereas the end-users of these technologies are called home teleconsumers or home telepatients. HHT technologies include simple to complex avenues to electronic communications, such as the telephone, low- and high-speed video, audio recordings, CD-ROM, the Internet, and patient monitoring devices.

House calls are making a comeback, as are the primary care providers who made them. The difference is that house calls are now electronic. Their benefits are consistently recognized by those healthcare providers and consumers who have actually used them. Many healthcare strategists believe that the future of the home healthcare industry will require more applications of HHT. The biggest challenge is balancing the cost of service with the quality of care.

This chapter focuses on the state of telecommunications in the home and its applications to the health of these patients. A brief overview of changes in health culture provides the backdrop for many applications of HHT. Initially, HHT pioneers addressed the most costly chronic diseases. Those who are chronically ill want to be at home, if possible, and participate in personal and family activities of daily living to the fullest extent possible. All of which are becoming more possible through the use of HHT.

Services being provided for home patients to improve outcomes and reduce costs are presented under existing applications. Point-of-care systems provide comprehensive services that track things such as patient care, treatment outcomes, and costs. Five of these systems are reviewed. Emerging applications of HHT appear in the areas of chronic conditions and diseases, such as cancer, infirmity in the elderly, movement disorders, asthma, and physically challenged individuals.

Finally, problems in determining HHT benefits are discussed from the perspective of research design.

HEALTH CULTURE CHANGE

Healthcare in America has undergone drastic changes, and more changes are coming. New movements and mandates toward primary care, managed care, outpatient surgery, preventive medicine, capitation, and the informed patient have impacted our health culture beyond all expectations, resulting in a paradigm shift from program-centered care to patient-centered care. With a managed care dominated environment, hospitals are no longer the source of medical care power, decision-making, and influence that they once were. They are rapidly becoming merely another patient care resource used only for specific treatment purposes. Primary care physicians are once again at the hub of patient management, and the challenges facing them require new HHT solutions, thereby resurrecting the all-important house call.

Based on the educational principle of readiness to learn, when the education process takes place in the home, knowledge is more likely to be applied. This occurs not only because of the readiness to learn, but also because of the immediate proximity of the application and the reinforcement.

Before the mid-19th century, hospitals were on the fringe of medicine, and they were usually considered to be places of poverty, pestilence, and death. By the beginning of the 20th century, hospitals had become the hub of high-tech medical care. The shift away from the physician's office and the use of house calls to hospital-based care was reinforced by research, rapid technical advances, federal funding, and the emergence of medical specialties. With increasing demands on family physicians leading to fewer house calls, many patients felt abandoned. Healthcare became somewhat fragmented, lacking coordination and transferable patient information. Eventually the evolution of high-tech inpatient medicine made it easier to use pharmaceuticals and diagnostic tests to effectively manage patients with complex conditions. This enabled primary care physicians to once again assume more direct responsibility for the care of their patients.

With the advent of cost containment and managed care, nourished by improvements in the standards of care, the role of primary care physicians is settled. And far more of them are needed to support the transition to home healthcare. Hospitals are being downsized or closed at alarming rates, and many are converting primarily to outpatient services. Others are becoming specialty centers, and others are extending their reach into the community through the use of HHT applications.

Currently, primary care physicians are effectively treating most of their patients' problems without referral. When necessary, they become care coordinators by working directly with patients, the families, and other members of the treatment team to establish partnerships toward maximizing mutually agreed-upon goals. Such partnerships, which prevent and manage health problems, have become mandates of healthcare reform.

Communication is the key to successful change. Patient education, informed consent, established treatment goals and realistic expectations, and the evaluation of outcomes are essential to promoting health partnerships, which HHT can facilitate. However, one must be aware that there is no magic in telecommunications, and it cannot stand alone.

Among the essential considerations for applying HHT are the needs, habits, and attitudes of both providers and patients. Comfort and familiarity are crucial to ensuring the effective use of any new technology. This involves training the elderly to communicate more through the use of high-tech/high-touch technology. Ultimately, future generations will demand such services because of their familiarity with the technology. It is unrealistic to assume this change will happen overnight. From all indications, telepartnering between healthcare providers and patients is perhaps the most untapped resource and provides the greatest challenge to the use of telecommunications in the home.

Home healthcare is increasingly becoming part of the equation to control costs, reward shorter hospital stays, and empower patients to assume more responsibility in managing their own health problems and risks. Efforts to bring HHT to the general population must reflect an acute awareness of the idiosyncrasies of care providers, consumers, and payers. Those living in rural or underserved areas will be the biggest beneficiaries as long as the technologies used are cost effective and accessible. Above all, telecommunication applications must meet home healthcare needs and be capable of adjusting to change. Areas of home healthcare that need further exploration for potential HHT applications are preventive care, acute care, post-acute care, long-term care, and hospice care. Ideally, each application should have both immediate and long-term cost benefits. The home healthcare culture will continue to change as users become more familiar and comfortable with HHT applications.

HHT APPLICATIONS

There is a growing population of people in the United States with chronic diseases, representing the vast majority of annual personal healthcare costs. The number of Americans requiring constant home healthcare will expand dramatically as the "baby boomers" age. HHT applications can be categorized into three groups: existing applications, point-of-care systems, and emerging applications. It is no surprise that the industry initially focused on costly common chronic illnesses, such as coronary heart disease, diabetes, and cancer, followed by other less costly health problems and issues (Figure 4–1).

FIGURE 4–1

Existing HHT Applications*	
Coronary Heart Disease	Cardiac Monitoring
	Rehabilitation
	Information Support
Diabetes	Glucose Monitoring
	Nutrition and Exercise
	Other Self-help Services
Cancer	Home Infusion Therapy
	Support Services
Other Health Problems/Issues:	
Health Promotion, Emergencies	Information Support
Osteoarthritis, Alzheimer's Disease	Patient Education
Cessation of Tobacco Use	Reminders
Medical Compliance	Monitoring
Appointment Making/Keeping	Counseling

*Telephone/computer-based services.

Sources: E. Andrew Balas, Farad J., Gilad J.K., et al: Electronic Communication with Patients, Evaluation of Distance Medicine Technology, *JAMA* 278(no. 2), 1997, pp. 152–159; Ron J. Pion, Portnow J.M., et al: Trends in Home Health Care: Past, Present, and Future, Interviews with the Experts, *Home Care Consultant* 1(no. 1), 1994, pp. 6–21; Glenn Edwards: The Untapped Potential of Home Health Care, *Journal of Health Care Benefits* July/August 1992, pp. 34–37.

EXISTING HHT APPLICATIONS

Coronary Heart Disease

More than one out of four living Americans will die from heart disease even though major advances have been made both in its management and prevention. The rising incidence of heart disease death rates reflects an aging population. Much like diabetes, heart disease requires moderate to drastic changes in lifestyle. The risk factors alone provide many opportunities to facilitate behavior modification efforts through HHT. At the very top of the list of HHT applications for heart patients is monitoring, nutrition, and exercise. Patients can now be monitored on a 24-hour basis for cardiac events within their homes. Projected financial savings from providing such daily HHT services are persuasive. Moreover, millions of people using home healthcare for other illnesses also have heart problems. In looking at HHT applications in the area of heart disease; cardiac monitoring, recovery from heart problems, and information support are the most obvious.

Cardiac Monitoring

Cardiac monitoring in the home is rapidly becoming a common practice for patients with certain types of arrhythmia. This practice allows unusual cardiac events to be detected and tracked. A device is worn that records abnormal heart palpitations or irregular beats when activated by the patient. The recording can be subsequently transmitted over the telephone (transtelephonic) directly to the physician. Patients can immediately receive assurances from their physicians by telephone that they are safe. The payoff is better diagnoses, fewer ER or ICU visits, better accuracy, and increased cost effectiveness. Several types of monitoring devices, including the Heart Card™, provide an effective means of reducing fear and reassuring patients recovering from a recent heart attack or heart surgery.

Recovery

Recovery from cardiac problems is now being facilitated by several HHT applications that focus on changing patient lifestyles.

As with diabetes, lifestyle modifications include exercise and diet. Routine exercise sessions can be accessed in combination with EKG monitoring, all from the home.

Patients can interact with care providers at a central location in addition to other patients participating in the home-based cardiac recovery programs. Several benefits are recognized by patients who use group support. Patients merely sharing their coping experiences is often an effective means of reducing anxiety, fostering confidence, and promoting physical activity. The therapeutic and social benefits of patients just becoming friends are also a bonus. Such support services are not only cost effective, they improve patient compliance and satisfaction. HHT offers patients the benefits of group support and social interaction without having to leave home.

Information Support

Information support is available through many HHT resources. Computer-based program packages enable patients to plan and track their diets, access shopping lists, and print out support materials.

The Internet offers a vast array of Web sites, chat rooms, and other on-line services that collectively represents what could be termed a "heart network." The American Heart Association has a Web site that provides self-assessment tools for identifying risk factors, exercise information, and answers to commonly asked questions about the relationship between heart disease and menopause, diabetes, and hypertension.

Leaving home can be highly problematic for many cardiac patients in rehabilitation. HHT options also link hospital-based dieticians and nutrition educators with patients, resulting in low costs and high user satisfaction. Interactive voice response (IVR) systems, the use of touch-tone telephones, telephone reminders (usually for medications and appointments), and 24-hour access to care providers all help make the ordinary telephone the backbone of HHT support for coronary heart disease.

Once again, HHT applications reach patients in an environment where their readiness to learn is optimal and their use of knowledge is immediate and practical.

Diabetes

Diabetes affects between 13 to 15 million Americans and only half of them even know they have this potentially life-threatening chronic disease. Diabetes management requires routine glucose monitoring and lifestyle modification. In the absence of such an effort, diabetics are more likely to experience routine hospital visits, debilitating conditions, and early death. Major complications associated with diabetes include heart disease, renal failure, amputations (as a result of poor circulation and repeated infections), neuropathy, retinopathy, and all too often, blindness.

The cost of managing diabetes is more than $100 billion annually. Both the incidence and costs will undoubtedly continue to grow as a function of increased life expectancy in combination with a growing population that will develop age-onset diabetes. Because diabetes is a chronic disease that is among the most amenable to self-help, the potential for HHT to assist patients in monitoring and managing glucose blood levels alone is extensive. Services that can be provided to diabetics at home include glucose monitoring, nutrition and exercise information and counseling, reminders, and self-help diabetes management information.

Glucose Monitoring

Glucose monitoring is considered to be a major breakthrough in diabetes management. Monitoring and maintaining blood glucose levels can effectively reduce the incidence of diabetic neuropathy and retinopathy to normal ranges. Many non-insulin diabetics do not monitor their blood glucose. The problem is similar to managing hypertension. The condition itself may remain silent, but the consequences may eventually become life threatening. This situation provides a major challenge to diabetes awareness and behavior modification.

Once the patient has been convinced of the long-range benefits of controlling blood glucose levels and has adopted habits to control it, HHT can provide support and refinement of the self-management process.

Many patients still prefer the manual approach to recording insulin readings even though sophisticated software packages are now in use that expand patients' level of self-management by graphing levels of blood glucose. With computer-compatible glucose measuring equipment, patients can now enter data, obtain answers to their questions through Web sites, and interact with healthcare providers to modify treatment plans—all within the home. Effective management of diabetes, particularly the regulation of blood glucose, requires constant vigilance and ongoing modifications in lifestyle, especially in regard to nutrition and exercise.

Nutrition and Exercise

Nutrition and exercise continue to be almost as important as glucose monitoring in the diabetics' efforts to control their disease. Effectively managing the triad of blood glucose, nutrition, and exercise is absolutely critical. Managing diabetes becomes a lifestyle, with common problems and solutions. HHT contributes to the process of establishing healthy diabetic lifestyles by offering practical solutions to common nutrition and exercise problems that fit the needs of the individual. Software is available that provides dietary and exercise information—including menus, recipes, weight management strategies, and nutritional and exercise facts and principles—geared toward disease management for diabetics and family members.

Nutritional counseling can be found on the Internet. The importance of exercise and its relationship to both nutrition and metabolism can be clarified through HHT-delivered information and chat rooms.

Regulating the disease is the biggest challenge for diabetics. The expanding role of HHT, including other self-help services on diabetes management, should make this effort much easier and more effective.

Other Self-Help Services

Other self-help services on diabetes are available through HHT. Telephone reminders have been used successfully in reducing serious podiatry problems. The fastest growing communication service for diabetics is the Internet, which offers a variety of information sources. Various organizations, such as the American Diabetes Association, maintain Web sites, chat rooms, and bulletin board services (BBSs) that address special information needs of diabetics. Reminders, role-playing, and information sharing are but a few of the growing options for diabetics through the major on-line services.

Cancer

Cancer is a complex disease that is often costly and difficult to manage. Most treatments are provided in an outpatient setting, including the home. The age of patients ranges from infants to the elderly. The diversity of patient needs in the management of cancer—augmented by different conditions, therapies, and patients—is challenging HHT developers. Cancer touches every aspect of life, frequently with strong emotional ramifications. The stigma of having cancer continues to plague patients, families, and friends.

HHT applications have facilitated the delivery of emotional help for cancer patients and families through support groups, chat rooms, and other on-line services. The establishment of Web sites by government, voluntary, and healthcare institutions to assist cancer patients and families through the treatment process has contributed to the process of validation and expansion of HHT use. The major on-line services offer comprehensive resources on cancer to their consumers.

Early HHT efforts toward cancer relied on the development of generic solutions that applied to common problems and needs in home healthcare for cancer patients. The use of home infusion pumps was among the first applications, followed by other electronically delivered support services.

Home Infusion Therapy

Home infusion therapy administers hydrating fluids, therapeutic drugs, nutritional products, and painkillers often in combination to cancer patients. They are reliable and quite simple to operate. Some pumps can be remotely regulated through the telephone or computer by physicians or pharmacists to meet individual patient needs. Pumps are physically manageable, tamper-proof, and designed to simultaneously deliver a variety of therapies and modes. With proper orientation, patients can acquire much more control over the management of their cancer through the use of home infusion pumps operated through HHT.

When using this type of technology, unfamiliarity and fear are once again overwhelming obstacles for some patients. Those who use the pump are generally more comfortable with their condition and are better able to participate in their therapy plan. Twenty-four-hour telephone monitoring of devices such as the home infusion pump has contributed to its effectiveness, expansion, and increasing levels of satisfaction among healthcare providers, patients, and third-party payers. One main use of the home infusion pump is to provide nutrition to cancer patients.

Improper nutrition is a major problem among cancer patients. Nutrition by infusion is sometimes necessary when undergoing therapies that may prevent eating. Infusion therapy can be fine-tuned to each patient's nutritional needs. The main advantage of infusion pumps is their ability to treat the patient at home. These patients tend to do better than those treated outside the home. The use of computer technology and the telephone to provide home infusion pump therapies is a major advance in home healthcare.

Support Services
The support services for cancer patients on the Internet are impressive. Major on-line services provide access to Web sites of the American Cancer Society and the National Cancer Institute. Other topical Web sites cover areas such as breast cancer, pediatric oncology, families of children with cancer, treatment options, and new developments in cancer research. Through a variety of on-line services, cancer patients can acquire assistance, information, and interactive support. Many healthcare professionals volunteer medical information, support, and referrals. Parenthetically, home healthcare users must be cognizant of the growing number of potentially harmful cancer remedies and cures that appear on the Internet.

Until the Internet became accessible, communication about cancer was limited to groups of researchers and practitioners who seldom talked to each other. Because direct-to-consumer advertising of healthcare products and services is expanding, it has been suggested that misinformation on the Internet may require policing. Some Web site developers claim that ridiculing those that post bad information is more effective than censoring them. In short, the accuracy of information is increasingly being challenged as more people have access to it. Ultimately, the long history of cancer treatment frauds can be combated by accurate and authoritative consumer information on the Internet and other HHT applications.

More traditional audio, video, and print materials supplement many of the Web sites. Interactive video technology has been used to communicate with home caregivers of pediatric cancer patients and provide for social interaction among older cancer patients.

One program uses two-way video for hospitalized patients to communicate with their family members at home. Reminder telephone calls and counseling have significantly improved the use of mammograms and other screening services. The balance of evidence suggests that the role of HHT in keeping many patients informed and enhancing their therapeutic communication is vital to the process of living with cancer.

Other Health Problems and Issues

Health promotions, emergencies, osteoarthritis, Alzheimer's disease, cessation of tobacco use, medical compliance, and appointment-keeping are among the other applications of HHT.

Except for health promotion computer networks, the majority of applications rely on touch-tone telephones in the home. Telephone reminders have been effectively used to improve elderly patients' use of immunizations, medication compliance, appointment-keeping, and preventive care procedures. Twenty-four-hour access to emergency consultations with home healthcare providers has reduced emergency room visits and hospitalizations. Ongoing telephone support has proven valuable in improving patients' emotional status and satisfaction with their care.

Interactive telephone systems using computer-based IVR systems enable users to obtain prerecorded messages or mini-lectures, make or change medical appointments, receive reminders, and obtain answers to common disease-specific questions. IVR systems are just as effective as printed questionnaires in obtaining health information and screening. Point-of-care systems provide a comprehensive means of capturing and organizing patient care data through the use of HHT.

POINT-OF-CARE SYSTEMS

Point-of-care systems (POCSs) are currently the most effective means of tracking and storing automated patient records between a central provider base and the home healthcare patient. Treatment plans, therapies, demographics, costs, and patient outcomes are among the data that POCSs can track. Accountability, cost effectiveness, and efficiency are driving forces in the structuring of POCS, which can vary in their scope and depth.

POCSs are rapidly becoming the common denominator of home healthcare delivery, quality assurance, and cost accounting. They empower healthcare providers, using a communication network, to partner with patients in delivering and adjusting treatments, informing, counseling, evaluating quality of care, and analyzing cost benefits. POCSs (or versions of them) may well be a valuable tool in the establishment and refinement of clinical protocols and treatment plans.

With capitation becoming the key to reimbursement, POCSs and other HHT systems provide the means by which mutually agreed-upon goals can be met while still maintaining the standards of care. The availability of POCS-generated data for evaluating the efficacy of treatments, including benefits, coupled with instant communication between care providers and patients should be particularly encouraging to those concerned with quality of care.

POCSs can be tailored to the needs of patients and will ultimately become a universal requirement in the home healthcare industry (Figure 4–2). Healthcare leaders recognize the benefits of POCSs in expanding the role of hospitals in the community. Some POCSs are clinically appropriate, although they are not always immediately cost effective or accessible. The ultimate goal is to expand the POCS concept to its capacity—the creation and support of healthy lifestyles that will reduce both human and financial costs.

FIGURE 4–2

Point-of-Care Systems*	
Home Assisted Nursing Network (HANC)™	Robot assistance (i.e., voice capability) for daily support, information, monitoring, and data entry over telephone lines
Medical Oriented Operating Network (MOON)™	IVR system for daily support, information, monitoring, data entry over telephone lines
The Personal Telemedicine System (PTS)™	Two-way interactive video visits for daily support, information, monitoring, and data entry over telephone lines
ResourceLink™	Two-way interactive television visits for daily support, information, monitoring, and data entry over local cable television lines
The Tevital Telehealth System™	Two-way interactive video visits for daily support, information, monitoring, and data entry over telephone lines and CD-ROM

*All Point-Of-Care Systems have a central nursing station.

Sources: HANC network, HealthTech Services Corp., Northbrook, IL; MOON, Unitron Medical, Clearwater, FL; PTS, American TeleCare, Eden Prairie, MN; ResourceLink, HELP Innovations, Inc., Lawrence, KS; Tevital Telehealth System, Tevital Inc., Paoli, PA.

POCSs are designed to provide 24-hour access, ease of use, cost savings, and versatility. All HHT applications are fluid; that is, they are affected by rapid changes within the healthcare and telecommunications industries. POCSs must remain generic and flexible in order to respond to such changes.

Facilitating disease management programs with POCSs is a winning proposition for care providers, consumers, and payers. Reductions in inpatient and outpatient visits, travel, and emergencies are among the many advantages of POCSs. Only long-range financial benefits may have to be acceptable before widespread use of POCSs will occur in all potential areas of service. Given the perceived value of POCSs, access and costs continue to hinder their expansion. Their cost benefits must be substantiated. Whatever the application, HHT must foster patients' confidence in their welfare and safety at home.

The following text describes five POCSs, which will be reviewed by their requirements, features, and benefits.

The Home Assisted Nursing Network (HANC)™

Several years ago, the HANC was described as an FDA-approved robot designed and programmed to assist home patients with their daily health needs.[1]

Requirements

The requirements include the placement of computer-like equipment in the patient's home, from which it is voice-linked to a central nursing station for assisting, prompting, and monitoring the patient's daily activities over regular telephone lines. The 42-inch-tall robot has a video screen and voice for assisting, prompting, and monitoring the patient's daily activities. Monitoring devices such as a thermometer and blood pressure cuff can be attached.

One central nursing station supported up to 50 HANC robots, monitoring and collecting patient information on a 24-hour-a-day basis. Nurses were prepared through an eight hour training program using the "training-the-trainer" concept. Nurses learned how to use the proprietary software to control care delivery, collect data, and create reports for physicians and third-party payers. HANC itself trained patients through its audio and video programming, walking them through a range of procedures.

Features

The features of HANC include diabetes management, wound care, infusion therapy, medication instructions and other directives, and monitoring vital signs and daily activities. Among the unique features of HANC is its voice capability, which directs patients (e.g., "It's time to take your medication."), provides encouragement (e.g., "That's all right, take your time."), and helps solve problems (e.g., "How can I help you?").

As a personal assistant, HANC can be programmed to provide reminders, prompt and coach patients, collect data, alert the central nursing station, monitor and modify treatment, and verbally communicate (it is multilingual) in a voice selected by the patient.

HANC's troubleshooting capabilities have proven to be highly effective. For example, parents with sick children having problems with a ventilator were assisted by HANC to apply corrective procedures or summon assistance from the central nursing station. Some families using HANC were initially apprehensive. Once it was functioning within their homes, patients and families became excited and pleased with the capabilities of HANC.

Benefits
Benefits include HANC's capability to address specific home healthcare needs in diabetes management, wound care, and infusion therapy—all at significant cost savings. Although unit costs initially ranged from $10,000 to $20,000 and central nursing units cost about $7,000, cost benefits were significant when home nursing visits could be avoided. A less costly version of HANC has emerged in the form of the CareMonitor.

Medical Oriented Operating Network (MOON)™

MOON is a telecommunications network that transmits data from the home to central nursing station providers, who track, manage, and coordinate the patient's care 24-hours-a-day.

Requirements
The requirements are flexible and have several home hardware options, including the regular touch-tone telephone, Minitel equipment, the "smart" device, and laptop computers with proprietary software. Touch-tone telephones are most frequently used. About 50,000 patients can be monitored by one electronic nursing station. If needed, video capabilities are also available for healthcare providers to confer with patients.

Little training is required for both patients and care providers to use the MOON. The patient is prompted through a simple IVR menu with instructions or questions. Both patients and providers use identification numbers to access patient records to ensure confidentiality and accuracy.

Features
The features of MOON include IVR programs that solicit data that are transmitted in real time and entered into the patient's

digital medical record at the central nursing station. This provides up-to-the-minute information, such as is usually required for inpatients. At the time of discharge from the hospital, the clinical healthcare team establishes a home treatment plan, which is entered into the patient's database in addition to lab results, histories, imaging, and other data. MOON can reduce the length of stay while extending the length of care more effectively. Furthermore, MOON is virtually a bridge from the hospital (or electronic nursing station) into the patient's home, with many of the same benefits as the hospital, particularly the continuity of care. This tends to make physicians more comfortable with earlier discharges. Perhaps the biggest contribution MOON has made is to figuratively extend the walls of the hospital following the discharge of patients. Physicians find the coordination of care through use of the MOON to be less fragmented, higher in quality, and more cost effective.

MOON is a simple, accessible approach to home healthcare. It requires no special equipment and can operate in eight different languages. Patient and provider entries are instantly captured on-line, allowing care providers to monitor the patient's condition and access medical records in combination with the treatment plan. Alerts appear when patients need follow-up home care or triage. Healthcare providers can order and track requests for things such as services, facilities, equipment, and pharmacy. Even healthcare providers are tracked to confirm home visits. Authorized users can access current patient records at any time. Diabetes monitoring, wound management, and orthopedics are the most prevalent applications of MOON, while others are currently being tested. The potential of the MOON appears to be limitless. It could easily be expanded to other areas of daily living for homebound patients.

Benefits

The benefits of MOON are its accessibility, versatility, and low cost. There is a monthly patient fee, including the Minitel charting device, that is charged for all services on an unlimited basis. Healthcare providers do not pay to use MOON. Equipment costs for establishing a central nursing station range from $75,000 to $150,000. Its capacity to provide immediate service to the patient at home at little cost and with minimal training of providers and patients makes MOON a viable and attractive alternative in HHT.

The Personal Telemedicine System (PTS)™

PTS allows two-way interactive video visits between the patient and nurse over regular telephone lines.

Requirements

The requirements include a PTS home unit, about two feet square, with a 2½-inch square color video screen, a camera, a microphone, a telephone, and attachments. The second version of the PTS unit is a PC based system with a 14-inch square screen. Attachments provide certain diagnostic and monitoring functions, such as taking the blood pressure, providing close-up views of wounds, and assisting with insulin syringe measurements. Color-coded buttons can be programmed for these applications. Providers have a similar unit to communicate with patients in addition to a separate receiving device for patient-transmitted information.

On the average, one hour is required to prepare home patients to use the system. Depending on the number of applications needed, 3 to 4 hours of training is needed by providers to operate the system. Providers are also prepared to select and train patients.

Features

The features of PTS capitalize on the self-management approach to home healthcare, in which a variety of uses are evident. Applications initially focused on elderly patients living alone, post-operative patients, dialysis and infusion therapy patients, AIDS patients, and those patients living in remote rural areas where direct home healthcare services are lacking. Other patient needs are met through routine PTS video contact between the patient and the nurse.

PTS delivers many of the routine services of the home-visiting nurse; including medication modifications, wound assessment, neurological evaluation, and frequent reminders and assistance for elderly patients with heart disease, dementia, or chronic obstructive pulmonary disease (COPD). PTS delivered patient education and counseling has proven to be effective in solving many problems in the self-management of conditions requiring patient initiative and compliance. Electronic charting and scheduling are also possible with supplemental software.

Benefits
The benefits of PTS can be attributed to its simplicity, versatility, immediacy, and accessibility. The basic home unit is $3,900 per year or $10 per day when rented, and it requires only a common telephone jack. The cost to equip the central nursing station is $3,000 to $8,000, depending on the software integration with patient tracking and triage programs. Some patients even dress and groom themselves for their video visits. For those patients living alone or in remote areas where home healthcare is seriously limited, PTS may be a welcome alternative in preventing loneliness and depression.

ResourceLink™

ResourceLink, developed by HELP Innovations, Inc., provides two-way interactive television visits between patient and nurse over regular cable television lines—the TV house call.

Requirements
The requirements for equipment include a 13-inch color television monitor with an attached video camera strategically located in the patient's home. Attachments are also available to examine heart and lung sounds. There are no knobs or buttons on the patient's monitor. The care provider is equipped with a personal computer, a monitor with "picture-in-picture" capacity, a video camera, and headset. Patients simply sit in front of their special television and camera during the entire TV house call and observe the nurse on the screen. No training is required for the patient to use ResourceLink. When a TV visit is scheduled, the patient merely sits in front of the television monitor. Providers are trained in televised patient care through a special course.

Features

The features of the unit include a 30 video frames per second picture, no buttons or knobs, automatic alerts from attached patient monitoring devices, and non-medical visit options with friends and family members. Two minutes prior to the scheduled TV visit, a beep is sounded and the set automatically turns on. ResourceLink services cover a broad range of chronically ill patients, including COPD, congestive heart failure, diabetes, high blood pressure, and terminal conditions. Specific applications include assistance in changing wound dressings, monitoring medication and activities of daily living, and educating patients.

One of the most impressive features is ResourceLink's capacity to address the patient's clinical and social needs. Many patients bond with their ResourceLink provider and find the multiple weekly visits to be extremely helpful in carrying out procedures and providing much-needed social interaction, particularly among patients who live alone. Many examples of success have been documented with the use of ResourceLink. For example, some patients have avoided nursing home placement, while others are better able to care for themselves and improve the quality of their life as a homebound patient.

Benefits

The benefits of ResourceLink encompass a variety of clinical and social needs of home healthcare patients. The capability of ResourceLink to assist homebound patients through self-management procedures while fostering what generally becomes a highly supportive relationship between the provider and the patients, has proven to be highly effective. The patient unit costs around $5,000 depending on attachments. Nursing unit costs are based on the number of patients covered. A single patient can be visited using ResourceLink up to four times a day at half the cost of one in-person house call. Additional applications of ResourceLink are being considered in the areas of mental health, physical and occupational therapy, speech therapy, and other non-medical visits.

The Tevital Telehealth System™

The Tevital Telehealth System is a two-way interactive video system with attachments that uses regular telephone lines for patient/nurse home video visits and has CD-ROM capabilities.

Requirements

The requirements include a small workstation housing a color television screen up to 15 inches in size. It has only five large buttons (thus avoiding the look of a computer) that interface with the video screen. The home workstation has a CD-ROM drive that provides information specifically selected for the patient's particular condition. Patients do not control the Tevital Telehealth System—they interact with it and a central nursing station provider.

The provider is located at a central nursing station with two video screens. One screen has picture-in-picture capacity so that the nurse can be seen by the patient while the other screen displays patient data. The nurse controls the patient's camera, which can capture images at high-resolution and store them in the patient's record.

Little patient training is necessary. They are prompted throughout the entire care process. When required, the Tevital Telehealth System can operate on its own. Providers must complete 3 to 5 days of training on the use of electronic patient records, electronic patient information retrieval, and the video visit itself.

Features

The features of the Tevital Telehealth System focus on the elderly patient. All of the interactive components are designed to accommodate frail older patients. Functions include patient assessment, medication monitoring and compliance, patient education, and crisis intervention. Ancillary educational opportunities are provided to maximize the patient's involvement in his or her own care. The developers appear to have made a concerted effort to make the system extremely practical, quality-driven, and user-friendly. Nurses routinely send instructions on taking medications and checking vital signs, provide care assistance, and review patient transmitted data via video.

Among other features of the Tevital Telehealth System are prompting and recording the patient's use of medications, archiving all patient records (including video visits), transmitting multimedia information for storage and future use, and providing clips of video visits to distant relatives when requested.

Benefits

The benefits are particularly evident in providing home healthcare for older patients. In many cases the Tevital Telehealth System has prevented the need for hospitalization, admission to skilled nursing facilities, and live-in assistance. The cost is $8,200 for the patient unit and $19,000 for each nursing unit. One nursing station can serve from 12 to 15 patient units. The cost per video visit is about one quarter of the charge for an actual home healthcare nurse's visit.

EMERGING HHT APPLICATIONS

Patient groups in need of more home healthcare services are the elderly and patients with chronic diseases and conditions and infectious autoimmune diseases (Figure 4–3).

Because of aging populations and the expanding role of patients, opportunities for innovative HHT applications appear to be unlimited. The three areas noted above present difficult, long-term healthcare challenges. Because many of these patients will not improve, emphasis should be placed on quality of life within their own home. Many HHT applications have already proven to be better equipped to meet certain home healthcare needs at less cost than traditional means. The mission of healthcare providers is to expand on current successes. We are merely looking at the tip of the iceberg of home healthcare needs that can be met in part by HHT applications. Perhaps the single largest high-priority population is the elderly.

The Elderly

The elderly represent the fastest growing population in the United States. The number of seniors in the "oldest old" segment

FIGURE 4–3

Emerging HHT Applications	
Elderly and Underserved	Mental Health Services
	Medication Compliance
	Wellness Programs
	Psychiatry
Chronic Conditions:	
Arthritis, Asthma,	Information Support
Sinusitis, Dermatitis,	Patient Education
Hay Fever, Hypertension,	Compliance
Migraine Headache,	
Orthopedic Impairments	
Autoimmune Diseases	Infusion Therapy
	Psychiatry
	Patient Education

Sources: Marshall Rockwell, Pion, R.: Medicine in the Year 2005: A Step into the Future, *The Remington Report*, August/September 1994, pp 7–10; Harry Fini: New Technologies Assist Health Care Providers, *The Remington Report*. August/September 1994, pp. 18-21; Arthur E. Schiller: Building the New Home Health Information Infrastructure, *The Remington Report*, August/September 1994, pp. 25–27.

are expanding more rapidly than any other group, and their health status can be extremely variable. Over 85% of non-institutionalized elderly patients suffer from at least one definable chronic medical condition, representing a large potential for home healthcare.

Because the elderly are living longer, which adds to the number of patients with co-morbidities, the need for more home healthcare alternatives is strikingly apparent. Given the large number of older patients, including those who are frail and prefer to stay in their homes, the challenge is to facilitate home healthcare in the most cost-effective manner possible using HHT. Prerequisites to this effort are patient independence, quality of care and life, and cost benefits. With the increasing ability through new medical technologies to extend the lives of those with chronic illnesses, total cost containment may not be possible. This only adds to the incentive to do more for less, when possible, within the patient's home.

With many chronic illnesses, improvements are reflected by short- and long-term benefits. HHT can promote such benefits through reductions in on-site personnel and costly office or emergency room visits and hospitalizations.

Mental Health Services

Mental health services are needed by increasing numbers of elderly patients. The long, successful history of the use of two-way interactive video to provide psychiatric treatment is a compelling force in home healthcare. With the establishment of POCS and other HHT applications, the dearth of geropsychiatric nurses can be optimized. One POCS nurse can manage up to 15 patients a day, whereas the same nurse might be able to visit in-person up to only four patients per day, based on the distances that must be traveled. The management of depression—the most common mental disorder among the elderly—can be accomplished effectively through video-based interactive psychiatric programs.

Video visits have proven to be highly effective in meeting the mental health needs of elderly patients, particularly those who live alone. The patient's anticipation of and preparation for the video visit itself appear to have immense therapeutic value. The balance of evidence suggests that video visits for mental health problems and 24-hour access to professional support by telephone reduce over-utilization of healthcare providers and unnecessary visits to the emergency room.

Patients who have undergone a severe heart attack or invasive procedure for heart disease often experience anxiety and depression. Follow-up counseling over the telephone has proven very effective in helping these patients through physical and psychological adjustments, in addition to alerting healthcare providers of any related problems requiring additional hospitalization.

Medication Compliance

Medication compliance among infirm older patients is a major factor in keeping these individuals at home and out of inpatient facilities. The management of this problem is multifaceted and has many pitfalls. The difficulties range from the patient's inability to read the labels and directions to the patient's beliefs that taking drugs does not really help. The cost of these patients not taking their medications is extensive. The use of telephone reminders alone may make a significant impact on reducing these costs.

Wellness Programs

Wellness programs focus on assisting the elderly in keeping physically active, eating properly, and maintaining their social life. This triad of wellness requires more HHT applications specifically tailored to infirm elderly patients. Mental disorders like depression, dementia, alcoholism, and bereavement often affect an elderly person's nutritional intake. For example, anorexia is a common symptom of depression among the elderly. While many patients do benefit from meal planning, certain elderly patients would benefit more from mental health services related to their underlying problem.

The power of routine social contact provided through patient–nurse or patient–patient video or audio visits should not be underestimated. Many elderly patients claim that the social benefits of routine telecommunication visits are extremely important to their well-being.

Chronic Conditions

Approximately 100 million people in the United States suffer from at least one chronic disease or condition. The most frequently seen are arthritis, asthma, chronic sinusitis, dermatitis, hay fever, heart disease, hypertension, migraine headaches, and orthopedic impairments. Current HHT applications address some of these conditions and diseases; however, they are mostly emerging areas.

More hospitals and medical centers are expanding their services to home healthcare through HHT applications, which has direct benefits to the hospital because of immediate service fees and subsequent patient hospitalizations. From Boston to California, institutional providers are attempting to follow their patients into the home to meet the requirements for continuity of care. Some providers are establishing POCSs, while others are limiting their efforts to smaller venues, such as the regular telephone.

Autoimmune Diseases

Over one million men, women, and children in America are infected with the HIV virus, which causes AIDS. Although there is still no cure, AIDS is approaching a new threshold in disease management. Combination drug therapies for many patients are effective in reducing the virus in the blood to undetectable levels. Because these new drug therapies require "by-the-minute" compliance, medication reminders are often vital to achieving desired outcomes.

The three areas of AIDS care that appear most appropriate for HHT applications are infusion therapy, psychiatric counseling, and patient education.

Infusion Therapy

Infusion therapy for AIDS patients represents a major portion of the infusion therapy industry. Home infusion therapy has been delivered to many AIDS patients at a cost savings of nearly 90%.

Home and hospice care provides both emotional and financial relief for a disease that is extremely costly. The telephone plays a very important role in the life of most AIDS patients.

Psychiatric Support

Psychiatric support includes routine counseling and support for AIDS patients. Even though the emphasis has now shifted from dying with AIDS to living with AIDS, the mental health needs of patients are still just as great. Re-entering the community, going back to work, having a social life, and becoming more physically active are common areas that require attention. More HHT applications are required to disseminate much-needed information on self-care and provide emotional support.

Patient Education

Patient education is the most active area of HHT applications for AIDS. AIDS-related information on the Internet alone represents the largest single effort to date devoted to a health problem. Numerous Web sites provide on-line materials, help lines, and databases to assist patients, families, and the general public. Bulletin boards and chat rooms are a vital resource for delivering late-breaking news, results of up-to-date research, and information exchange.

In general, HHT applications demonstrate the same benefits for AIDS patients as for other chronic diseases. In essence, HHT has the potential to meet many of the multiple needs resulting from AIDS in a more cost-effective manner.

BENEFITS OF HHT APPLICATIONS

The documented benefits of HHT applications are highly idiosyncratic and primarily anecdotal, as reported throughout this chapter. Much of the reason for this can be attributed to the lack of rigorously applied research and evaluation methodologies. Defining the research parameters, sampling, and controlling intervening variables are major problems in evaluating HHT outcomes. The absence of national home healthcare standards and treatment guidelines for many long-term or complex medical conditions are additional compromising factors. Furthermore, cost analyses are not standardized, thus preventing any significant comparisons between HHT applications and traditional care.

In reviewing the literature, there are few controlled studies that consistently demonstrate the same benefits in patient outcomes and costs from HHT applications. This could be due in part to incompatible research protocols. Nevertheless, some relatively common discernible benefits include high patient satisfaction, improvements in certain clinical outcomes, and fewer in-person medical visits and hospitalizations. Far more research using experimental or quasi-experimental designs is needed to substantiate the benefits of applications in HHT.

CONCLUSION

HHT is in its infancy and it must learn to crawl before walking. Far more effort is required in refining HHT applications, defining anticipated outcomes, and conducting valid and reliable evaluations. Areas in need of further study include the clinical, logistical, personal, and financial benefits of HHT. It is quite possible that HHT will ultimately fill the gap between inpatient and ambulatory care while establishing itself as a highly effective adjunct to home healthcare.

The opportunities for meeting home healthcare needs using telecommunications are limitless. As communication technology and networks evolve, HHT will eventually assist patients in ways never believed to be possible. The key is to develop applications that are accessible, useful, and make a significant difference in meeting healthcare goals. Successful HHT applications provide solutions to care problems that best facilitate patient outcomes and cost benefits.

REFERENCE

1. George Wiley: Technology's Future State, *Home Health Care*, May/June 1994, p. 84.

The New Screen Telephone

If consumer needs prevail, the new screen telephone will play a major role in the future of home health telecommunications (HHT). Current trends in the telecommunications industry favor the use of the telephone, especially since most consumers have one and are comfortable and familiar with its use. Because healthcare should not be delivered only to the privileged few, and the current costs of wiring America with broadband technology are prohibitive, the use of ordinary telephone lines will probably continue for many years. Using regular lines, the new screen telephone should be able to fill the time gap until it is financially viable to install a national broadband infrastructure that provides capabilities such as digital video communication to and from the home.

Among the major advantages of starting a national HHT effort using the new screen telephone are the following capabilities:

- Developing, testing, and refining patient programs
- Addressing new areas of patient care

- Evaluating the care management process
- Resolving hardware and service configuration issues

All this must be done while providing universal, accessible, cost-effective applications in home healthcare.

This chapter will identify some of the latest hardware in advanced screen telephony, including functions, marketing issues, and costs. The section on telephonic pathways, including frequently asked questions, addresses potential applications that the new screen telephone will bring to home healthcare. The capabilities of the new screen telephones to reduce both human and financial costs in home healthcare are discussed next. Finally, the implementation of the new screen telephone, which may require some education and training, particularly in the highly specialized areas of home healthcare, is discussed.

DISPLAY SCREEN TELEPHONES (SCREEN PHONES)

Manufacturers are capitalizing on the simplicity and familiarity of the telephone by developing telephones capable of higher communication levels than have ever before been reached. The evolution of the variety of telephone sizes and styles has included portable and wireless models. The first screen telephones had small liquid crystal displays (LCDs) that showed the dialed number and elapsed time of the call. Many of these phones can still be seen in the larger airports and other public areas. Later generations of display screen telephones (screen phones) also could display the number of the caller using Caller ID technology. However, these devices had small screens and were unsuitable for displaying significant amounts of textual material.

A new worldwide protocol, Analog Display Service Interface (ADSI), which was developed by Bellcore in 1993, allows the nearly simultaneous delivery of voice and textual information to a screen phone. For the first time, there is a standardized way for users to "see" information that heretofore was available only through audio means. In addition, the ADSI supports advanced call management services (ACMSs), such as call waiting, three-way calling, and call directories, and it provides a platform for other interactive applications, such as visual voice mail, home banking, stock quotes, and home healthcare. The ADSI protocol has significantly expanded potential access to databases through these new screen telephones.[1] The combination of these features has attracted attention for their potential to provide interactive on-line consumer services.

"ADSI provides service industries such as healthcare with a cost-effective, user-friendly means of communicating with their end user customers," says Tom Moresco, Director of Advanced Voice Services at Bellcore. "This can help increase the quality of customer care, while at the same time, reducing operational costs. Currently there are about 1.5 million ADSI screen phone owners in the United States and Canada. As with any mass market consumer technology, we expect that as the price of ADSI screen phones continues to drop, the deployment of ADSI-based products and services will expand and accelerate."[2]

Interactive voice response (IVR) systems provide touch-tone access to information (for example, when a person checks his or her bank balance or frequent flyer miles, or accesses a corporate phone directory). Screen phones offer visual prompts to information sources in the text on the screen and the familiar audio prompts. The user can touch either the appropriate key on the keypad or a "soft key" aligned with the text on the screen to enter his or her responses. As a result, the interaction may occur

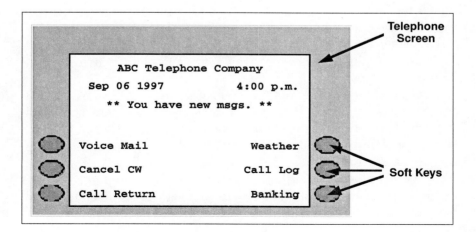

more rapidly because reading is generally faster than waiting for the voice prompts.

The newest version of screen phones represents a further breakthrough that enables users to communicate and access information. These Internet telephones provide access to the Internet, the World Wide Web (the Web), display text, and graphical information on the display screens—just like on a personal computer. This capacity is in addition to the comprehensive telephony functions built into these phones. Internet telephones offer great versatility by combining "smart" telephone capacity with Internet browsing and e-mail. Many see this advance as solidifying the future of the telephone.[3]

Categories of screen phones include the following:

- Screen phones that use Bellcore's ADSI protocol to provide advanced calling features, visual and audio prompts and access to databases (referred to as *screen phones* in this text)
- Screen phones that provide access to the Internet, retrieval of Web text and graphics, and support for advanced calling features (referred to as *Internet phones* in this text, even though they are essentially more advanced versions of generic screen phones)

Although ADSI screen phones can access the Internet for selected services, such as e-mail, information transfer speeds are relatively slow and the level of information is limited compared with the Internet or the Web. However, recent ADSI improvements have made it a very practical alternative for text-based e-mail communication. Internet phones integrate robust Web access and advanced calling features—a first in information technology.

There is a viable market for both low-end ADSI screen phones and high-end Internet phones, depending on the complexity of the information being exchanged between the health-care agency and the patient. Based on the assumption that a big future exists for both screen phones and Internet phones as high-tech replacement telephones that are complementing, not competing with, personal computers (PCs), several companies have entered the marketplace.

FIGURE 5–1

SUMMARY OF ADSI SCREEN PHONE FEATURES			
Product/Vendor			
AXIS	E-mail	Caller ID	Calendar
Uniden	Address book	On-hook dialing	Menu driven
	Keypad	Speakerphone	
CST-2100	E-mail	Caller ID	Directory
CIDCO	Address book	On-hook dialing	Keypad
	Call management	Adjustable screen	14 Soft keys
	Speakerphone	Menu driven	
PowerTouch 450	E-mail	Caller ID	Directory
Nortel	Address book	On-hook dialing	Keypad
	Call management	Adjustable screen	6 Soft keys
	Speakerphone	Menu driven	
Philips 980	E-mail	Caller ID	Directory
	Address book	On-hook dialing	Keypad
	Call management	Adjustable screen	Soft keys
	Speakerphone	Menu driven	Calendar

THE MARKETPLACE

Several manufacturers in the United States and abroad are producing ADSI screen phones and Internet phones. These appear to be similar in hardware specifications, but they vary in function, marketing, and cost. They all include a small keyboard that can be removed from sight when it is not in use (Figures 5–1 and 5–2).

The functions of Internet phones vary more by their Internet and Web access capacity. Various technologies are used to bring pages down from the Web and transfer them into smaller screens. Internet service providers (ISPs) are also expanding their support of small-screen consumers through special servers and gateways. Open server design promotes the development of

FIGURE 5–2

SUMMARY OF INTERNET PHONE FEATURES			
Product/Vendor			
iPhone	E-mail	Internet browser	Graphical display
CIDCO/	Grayscale	Touchscreen	Keyboard
InfoGear	Serial ports	Call management	Caller ID
	Directories	Yellow/white pages	Speakerphone
	Address book		
Alcatel 2840/2850	E-mail	Internet browser (Java)	Graphical display
(Planned for 1999)	Color	Touchscreen	Keyboard
	Serial ports	Call management	Caller ID
	Directories	Yellow/white pages	Speakerphone
	Address book		
Vestel USA	E-mail	Internet Browser	Graphical display
(Planned)	Color	Touchscreen	Keyboard
	Serial ports	Call management	Caller ID
	Directories	Yellow/white pages	Speakerphone
	Address book		

new Internet phone applications in many areas, including home healthcare.

HOME HEALTHCARE APPLICATIONS USING SCREEN PHONES

Common home healthcare applications are presented in Figure 5–3. Common telephone functions that serve non-health needs can be translated easily into applications that support the home healthcare environment.

TELEPHONIC PATHWAYS

Industry Views

The views of industry leaders vary on the immediate and long-range future of Internet phones. Some are optimistic, while

FIGURE 5-3

SAMPLE HOME HEALTHCARE APPLICATIONS USING SCREEN PHONES	
Phone Function	**Home Healthcare Applications**
Appointment-making	Office/home visits
Automatic callback	Reducing communication barriers*
Automated directions	Self-assessment/care
Call forwarding/waiting	Access/safety
Community bulletin boards	Health information transfer
Electronic white pages	Reducing communication barriers
Home banking/shopping	Nutrition planning/food purchasing
Pay-per-view	Accredited professional education
Time/temperature	Compliance/temperature control
Three-way calls	Patient conferencing/counseling
Redial	Reducing communication barriers
Stock quotes/corporate information	Home healthcare standards/policies
Visual voice mail	Care instructions/reminders
Voice mail access/control	Access/safety

*Ease of use particularly benefits patients who are physically or mentally challenged.

others believe the competition from TV-based Internet access may slow down mass acceptance of Internet phone technology. Tests are underway in various parts of the country in thousands of households. Initial applications include access to local information, such as shopping sales, school information, and public service announcements, and e-mail. Providing for the translation of Web documents that can be viewed on the small Internet phone screen has been a big challenge for developers. In the meantime, home healthcare applications could possibly facilitate marketing efforts by establishing a presence and refining the technology to maximize mass consumer adoption of the Internet phone as a tool for daily living with existing access to health information and services.

The Yankee Group, a Boston-based research company, has identified four issues that vendors need to address in the Internet phone industry.[4]

Product Positioning

Because the Internet phone appears to consumers to be a cross between a regular telephone and PC, confusion exists as to its market. And it competes with various Internet platforms, such as PCs and low-cost TV-based devices. Vendors must emphasize the value of Internet phone functions, such as easy Web access, call management, and home healthcare in addition to marketing to those early adopting consumers who do not have other devices. In addition, the ergonomics (i.e., where this instrument should be placed, such as the kitchen versus the study) may be a key factor in customer acceptance.

Standards

A continuing problem is the "format war," where both hardware and service configurations are proprietary.

Pricing

Consumers must be convinced of the value of both ADSI screen phones and Internet phones, particularly when they may already have access to the Web through a PC or their television.

Distribution

Many dealers find it difficult to support Internet phones because of the difficulties in explaining and demonstrating their use. With the implementation of advanced call management services, retailing the Internet phone should become easier.

Many companies are forming alliances in the Internet phone race, such as InfoGear, which joined forces with seven industry leaders. Robert L. Diamond (former chairman of the board of CIDCO) claims that "telephones are basic to the flow of communications in our society, and the iPhone enhances this use by bringing the richness of the Internet to consumers. The InfoGear platform opens a new world to consumers by providing convenient access to all the services and information on the Web through a familiar, simple, and easy-to-use telephone."[5]

From information now available, it appears that Internet phones may initially be more acceptable when they play a highly important role in the life of the user. Home healthcare is indeed one of several areas where Internet phone applications can provide access to vital information, medical support, and safety—all toward improving quality of life.

FREQUENTLY ASKED QUESTIONS

The following text discusses some of the most frequently asked questions about Internet phones.[6]

What Do Internet Phones Look Like?

Internet phones are simple telephone-like devices with small familiar screens. Some are touch screens, while others use a combination of buttons or keyboards. Internet phones are generally compact and lightweight.

Who Will Buy the Internet Phone?

Internet phones are designed for residential and small office customers who want a state-of-the-art phone with low-cost Internet access. Manufacturers believe that both technical and non-technical users will purchase Internet phones because they provide an affordable, easy-to-use telephone in addition to being an Internet-ready device. A typical PC takes from 3 to 5 minutes to power up, load Windows™, and run the Web browser, while some Internet phones provide immediate one-touch Internet access in approximately 3 seconds.

How Big Is the Internet Phone Market?

Because about 95% of all homes have a least one telephone, and there are an average of 2.4 telephones per household, the current number of installed telephones is about 240 million. Approximately 40% of all households (35 to 40 million) in the United States own one or more PCs, and 33% have access to the Internet.

Market estimates for Internet phones range from 1.5 to 10 million by the year 2005, representing 2% to 7% of all U.S. households.

Are Internet Phones the Same as PCs?

The Internet phone is not a PC. PCs do computing and store data, and generally range in price from under $1,000 to $2,000. They support a wide range of peripherals and application software. The specialized nature of the Internet phone makes it more affordable than a PC to more consumers.

Studies indicate that consumers perceive PCs to be confusing, cumbersome, and costly, whereas the telephone is currently the most widely used information device. PCs are generally targeted for businesses or home offices. Internet phones are designed for residential customers. Internet phones will co-exist with PCs similar to the co-existence of microwave and conventional ovens—complimentary instead of competitive.

Are Internet Phones Network Computers?

Network computers will be used with the Internet to access application software that resides elsewhere (i.e., on a server). Internet phones are neither network computers nor scaled down PCs. They are the next generation of information access devices (a logical evolution for the modern telephone).

Proponents of the network computer want to offer a low-cost alternative to PCs. Target pricing for the network computer is comparable to Internet phones, although the target audience and intended use are vastly different. The most viable markets for the network computer are in business and education, not the home.

How Much Will Internet Phones Cost?

Vendors (e.g., telecommunications companies, Internet service providers, and content providers) will offer Internet phones for a nominal charge or even for free, much like cellular providers offer cell phones at no charge if users sign up for 1 to 2 years of subscription service. Initially, prices are expected to be in the $350 to $500 range, and they will likely come down further in price soon after their introduction.

What Peripherals Are Available?

Many Internet phones include optional ports that support a range of peripherals, including printers, bar code devices, and smart card or credit card readers. Other peripheral applications that are specific to home healthcare are possible.

What About Future Peripherals?

Enhancements for most Internet phones will be cordless and will include larger LCDs, two phone lines, color graphics, transaction automation, fax capability, paging, advanced call handling, queue management, scheduling capabilities, and faster modems.

What Are Viable Commercial ADSI Applications for Screen Phones?

Common commercial ADSI applications include access to news, weather, stock quotes, horoscopes, and shopping. Healthcare is a rapidly emerging new application area for ADSI.

Why Is ADSI Vital to Information and Service Providers?

The use of audio-visual information access devices is made possible by ADSI. The airline industry has capitalized on this function by directly marketing flight services. Information access can be tailored to the profile of the user.

What About Plans for ISDN-Based Internet Phones?

Many Internet phones use a flexible platform that can accommodate either a normal telephone line or an ISDN line. This platform is currently being used primarily by enterprises and telecommuters. As mass market demand increases, costs decrease, and delivery is simplified, Internet phones will eventually be based on ISDN or ADSL.

What About Two Phone Lines?

Most Internet phones currently offer only one phone line. Two phone line support is planned by many of the new models of the Internet phone.

What About Faster Modems?

Faster speeds are already available through cable and other devices. Internet phone manufacturers will also offer faster modems in response to consumer needs.

Why Are the Telecommunications Companies Interested in Internet Phones?

Internet phones provide a unique opportunity for local and long distance carriers to do the following:

- Increased Internet access
- Branding
- Bundled services
- Service lock-in strategies
- Advertising revenues

Telecommunications companies can customize the systems with their own logo, class features, interactive services, Web-page content, advertisements, and Internet access service. HHT applications can be added to most Internet phone features.

What About Training and Education?

Vendors provide complimentary training and education materials and services to most buyers.

POTENTIAL INTERNET PHONE APPLICATIONS

"The major drivers of cost and demand for healthcare resources today are the progressive, chronic diseases," according to John A. McChesney, Chairman and CEO of Patient Care Dynamics, Inc. "Among the greatest impacts that can be made through

HHT is coronary heart disease. By merely examining the disease process, the first opportunity is in patient education. Risk factors can be clearly identified that predispose an individual to a higher risk and an accelerated rate and progression of cardiovascular disease, including gender, age, blood cholesterol level, blood pressure, smoking habits, diabetes, diet, and exercise. The goal is to identify those at risk with screening tests, which can be easily done over the I-Phone. Upon identifying those at increased risk, various activities can be initiated and supported along with access to information to help them minimize or eliminate those risk factors that will preordain them to an accelerated progression of the disease."[7]

When several risk factors are clearly evident, suggests McChesney, the likelihood of nonsymptomatic disease rapidly accelerates. Such patients feel great and healthy even though they are overweight, smoke, do not exercise, and their blood pressure is too high. The ultimate challenge is to motivate people who don't feel sick to give up what often gives them the most pleasure. Finding solutions to modify behavior and reduce risk factors is the ultimate challenge facing HHT providers.[8]

In keeping with the previously stated pathfinding hint on patient compliance, HHT protocols that routinely promote and reward changes in behavior could be more effective than infrequent office visits. The medical community and third-party payers must recognize and support efforts to provide a service that has great potential for reducing morbidity and healthcare costs.

In looking at the other end of the heart disease continuum (i.e., cardiovascular rehabilitation), several non-technical barriers exist. An independent cardiac rehabilitation home therapy service center in a community can be in competition with physicians, clinics, and hospitals. Attempts to set up such services often run afoul of the economic interests of local professionals or find other forms of resistance within the healthcare delivery system, observes McChesney.[9]

The primary care physician, cardiologist, or the cardiac rehabilitation unit at the hospital must be included in the equation. The cooperation and consensus of these components are essential. Because they make the decisions on prescribing drugs and rehabilitation therapy, an effective approach is to partner with them in making decisions to use an independent service. The financial aspects of the service may be a crucial factor, particularly capitation. The final decision usually depends on the economic benefits for all parties involved.

"We believe," says Khalid Mahmood, MD, of American Telecare, "that home telemedicine has to go on ordinary telephone lines, because they are installed in every patient's home. And since care cannot be delivered partially or segmentally to only the privileged few, we need to [use] ordinary telephone lines. We need to provide this care to everyone. The basic system has a video telephone that provides 8 to 10 frames per second on a small screen. It has blood pressure and pulse equipment, and the telephonic stethoscope that preserves the quality of sound in an analog fashion over ordinary household telephone lines. To this basic system one can attach, on an as-needed basis, other devices for patients who have, for example, heart problems. If you want to do an EKG or pulse oximetry, which is very simple, you tell the patient to put a finger into the pulse oximeter and have them hold it in front of the screen so that nurse can read it from the other end. Our system is very inexpensive. It costs $3,900, which is about the price of one IV therapy pump. We believe that this can facilitate care of patients, [and] it can improve the quality of care by enhancing the availability of nurses to patients. We are also finding that it can reduce the cost of care."[10]

Internet phone applications that may have particular relevance to HHT are discussed in the following text.

Information Transfer

Information transfer (i.e., surveys using touch-screen response) is used for risk assessment, disease management, patient monitoring, adverse drug responses, and patient satisfaction. "Examples that are well known," observes Dennis Tsu, Vice President for Marketing of InfoGear Technology Corp., "include patients hooking up self-monitoring equipment and transmitting the results to their physicians at a remote healthcare facility. Monitoring which today may be limited to a transfer of data from an EKG, may extend to a video camera hookup in the near future. [The day] is not far off [when] a patient might have a continuous hookup to a monitoring device in their homes [that] would call out to the hospital once an hour or whenever certain trigger events occur."[11]

Accessing Health Information

"In terms of general information . . . the Internet and the Web are a reservoir of data for the average layperson . . . to find out more about any aspect of their health, nutrition, general health practices, vaccinations, insurance, etc.," observes Tsu, "As people recognize this resource and take advantage of it, this should lead to a smarter healthcare consumer. As early examples, there are many HMOs already operating extensive Web sites for exactly this purpose."[12]

"As a corollary to this general information, there can be specific campaigns [centered] around preventing certain diseases and epidemics in the population. For instance, certain discussion groups might be targeted for information about the latest HIV vaccines and treatments, or a veterans group might be given information about potential nerve gas exposure. The converse of outbound targeted information is providing very detailed, specific information on a Web site for those who want to come and visit it. An example might be a site about dengue fever for people traveling to Southeast Asia. At a more common level might be a site from a dental care company about oral hygiene."[13]

E-Mail

Many of the applications require access to e-mail. Much of the transfer of information in healthcare management relies on the ability of both patients and providers to interact routinely by e-mail. This option is extremely important in providing on-going therapy and responding to specific questions of patients.

Ordering Products and Services

"Lastly," points out Tsu, "are those patients who are in the recovery stages from an operation or an illness. Pharmacies can offer prescription renewal over the Web, speeding refills and decreasing errors in the processing. The ability of a doctor to monitor patients remotely might lead to an ability to discharge patients earlier without any risk to their health."[14]

Providing User-Specific Information

Patients can be prompted through the use of Internet phones to remember to take their medications, thereby improving compliance. Alerts, updates, and news on the latest developments in various areas of healthcare are available to users on a daily basis.

Because Internet telephones are relatively new in the marketplace, specific applications for the home health sector must be developed. Fortunately, there is a long list of successful, well-established IVR applications that can be easily modified for both screen and Internet phone platforms. Many of these IVR applications enhance patient services and do not replace them. The successful health-related computerized IVR applications include the following:[15]

- Use in smoking cessation programs
- Treating mild to moderate depression and obsessive-compulsive disorders
- Monitoring drinking patterns of alcoholics and non-alcoholics
- Scheduling appointments and personally tailoring instructions on medication use

PATIENT AND COST BENEFITS

Because home healthcare is becoming recognized as a highly appropriate alternative to costly traditional care, the "digital door" is opening. Finding a solution for further reducing home healthcare costs through HHT applications is the single biggest challenge facing those in the industry. The bottom line is that home healthcare is here to stay and is growing at a phenomenal rate with increasing support for reimbursement. The Health Care Financing Administration (HCFA) is currently supporting demonstration sites for HHT applications. Several HMOs have also launched local and regional projects to test the efficacy of electronically delivered home healthcare.

The cost of many of the telecommunications devices is still viewed as a major deterrent to making home healthcare digital. Reimbursement is the key to enabling HHT to crawl before it walks, which is essential to establishing its presence as another solution for reducing costs and improving patient and provider satisfaction. Nevertheless, the evidence that HHT will play an expanding role in reducing both the human and financial costs of home healthcare is compelling, although it is limited by a dearth of scientific studies.

HHT solutions range from using regular telephones for providing medical follow-up, counseling, reminders, and interactive support to using highly sophisticated computerized systems for delivering infusion therapy. Given the current status of HHT, which is now gaining momentum by demonstrating its ability to warrant reimbursement, the relatively inexpensive Internet phone may be the critical first step in bringing home healthcare into the year 2000.

HOME HEALTHCARE TELEPHONE USE

The Internet phone or screen phone currently appear to be the most obvious cost-effective and appropriate contribution to HHT for a variety of reasons, including the following:

- In reviewing the literature, the evidence is overwhelming in support of the use of the telephone in home healthcare as a means of reducing costs in outpatient, hospital, or other settings, requiring a relatively small investment in new equipment and personnel.
- The use of the telephone represents a relatively inexpensive way to introduce home healthcare to the direct benefits of information technology, starting with simple cost-effective applications and expanding to more sophisticated add-on devices and programs to optimize patient and cost benefits.

- The telephone is the most familiar and commonly used means of personal communication in the United States, and consumers should be quite comfortable with new applications of the telephone, such as Internet phone technology.
- The use of the telephone should be considered to be an investment in the future of home healthcare as one of many new solutions to care management and cost containment. It is simply a matter of figuring out the most appropriate applications for today and tomorrow that reward everyone involved.
- Based on the results of outcomes research focused on the medical effectiveness of different forms of healthcare delivery, the use of the telephone promotes better self-care among patients.
- Various demonstration projects using a variety of telecommunications devices to monitor and manage medical problems have substantiated the concept and benefits of HHT.
- The savings provided by HHT because of a reduction of office, emergency room, and hospital visits alone is compelling evidence. Additional savings can be identified on a case-by-case basis in addition to better care outcomes.
- Unless there is a consistent revenue stream (which is more likely to occur with a HCFA reimbursement plan), a large number of patients, extensive operations, and a wide range of services being offered, the more sophisticated HHT applications may require careful planning.
- Initially, patients residing in rural areas and all homebound patients are most likely to receive federal support for HHT applications. The use of the telephone in these areas is almost a mandate in regard to human and cost benefits.
- Education and training requirements for both providers and users vary among HHT applications. The providers need from a few hours up to several days of training for

most applications, including point-of-care systems. Patients usually require a few minutes to several hours, depending on which application is used.

EDUCATION AND TRAINING

Healthcare is rapidly moving toward a patient-centered global care model for case management. From the mix of care options, the home has become a preference among most patients. The potential for augmenting, refining, and containing the costs of home healthcare through telephony will only be realized when its benefits are acknowledged by all concerned groups. Professional and public education campaigns are needed to inform all parties about the human and cost benefits of HHT applications.

Leaders in technology have responded to the need for new telecommunications pathways to the home by developing new devices and new versions of old devices. With the arrival of digital telephones, a new frontier has emerged. Many people still fear the high-tech world, which has promoted the user friendly movement among device designers. Only a small minority of our population actually have modems. Unfortunately, there is a tendency to not use information systems, particularly computers and other high-tech devices, by individuals who find it difficult to adapt or make the transition. Simplifying the use of HHT devices will go a long way toward implementing various applications.

The training of providers in HHT applications can take from a few minutes to a few days. Extensive training has been avoided for two reasons. The most obvious one is to keep the device as simple and easy-to-use as possible to facilitate user compliance. The second reason is to avoid unnecessary costs.

CONCLUSION

Telephony is an integral part of our lives. Increasing HHT applications through the new telephone will require cooperation between the decision-makers in telecommunications and home healthcare. Several new pathways have been explored and mapped for expansion to the home healthcare community. Telephony is the first step in the HHT movement.

REFERENCES

1. *ADSI Primer,* Global ADSI Solutions, Inc., Morganville, N.J., 1996.
2. Personal communication with Tom Moresco, Director of Advanced Voice Services at Bellcore, Inc., October 1998.
3. *Frequently Asked Questions for ADSI Partners,* Global ADSI Solutions, Inc., Morganville, N.J., April 15, 1997.
4. *From Screen Phone to Internet Phone: Consumer Communications,* White Telecare, Eden Prairie, MN, 1998.
5. J. Greenway, ed:. *Seven Industry Leaders Support InfoGear Technology Platform for Consumer Internet and Web Access,* p. 2, Las Vegas, NV, January 10, 1997, InfoGear Technology Corporation.
6. *Frequently Asked Questions, iPhone,* CIDCO, Inc., Morgan Hill, CA, 1997.
7. Personal communication with John A. McChesney, Chairman and CEO of PatientCare Dynamics, Inc., Mason, OH, January 1997.
8. Ibid.
9. Ibid.
10. Personal communication with Khalid Mahmood, American Telecare, Eden Prairie, MN, January 1997.
11. Personal communication with Dennis Tsu, Vice President of Marketing for InfoGear Technology Corporation, Redwood City, CA, June 1998.
12. Ibid.
13. Ibid.
14. Ibid.
15. Ron J. Pion, Portnow, J.M., et al.: Trends in Home Health Care: Past, Present, and Future, Interviews with the Experts, *Home Care Consultant* 1(no. 1), 1994, pp. 6–21.

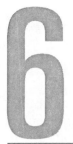

CHAPTER

The Telecommunications Industry and Healthcare

The merging of telecommunications and healthcare has created a new frontier of challenges and solutions. Added to the complexity of such combinations are the rapid changes taking place in the scientific and cultural aspects of medicine and healthcare delivery. It will require that new pathways be explored through collaborative efforts between telecommunications and healthcare providers and consumers.

This chapter begins by exploring a few of the main pathways of home healthcare telecommunications (HHT). Having already explored telephony in Chapter Two, the electronic patient record, the longitudinal health record, on-line networks, video, and television are among the remaining "prime movers" in the business of information transfer. Combining these telecommunications pathways into home healthcare applications, which requires solutions to common operational problems, is discussed from the perspective of the availability and cost-effective use of support services. HHT policy and cost issues leading to path building initiatives are presented, in part, through a series of questions answered by industry leaders.

CHALLENGES

The application of Diagnosis Related Groups (DRGs) and the increased ability to treat disease are resulting in earlier hospital discharges, which has led to a shift in expenditures for care in skilled nursing facilities and a rapid move toward home healthcare in an effort to reduce costs.

HELPFUL STRATEGIES

According to the Consumer Interest Research Institute, "Networks capable of bringing video and multimedia communications into and out of homes can provide a vast realm of new services, including:

- Knowledge and motivational methods to prevent illness and promote wellness
- Self-care information
- Easy consultation with healthcare professionals
- Sophisticated management of chronic diseases
- Support for convalescence from acute care
- Supervision and training for home care workers
- Support groups for patients with similar health conditions

In the long run, regular home health monitoring can take us to a new level of medicine with early detection of disorders and treatment customized to individual responses.

If we can utilize the information highway to deliver healthcare to the home, we can provide more cost effective and timely care . . ."[1]

Strategies for change focus on the following:

- Advancing and implementing telecommunications networks
- Developing an integrated patient record exchange system
- Removing financial disincentives through reimbursement

- Establishing awareness of the benefits of telecommunications in home healthcare

HOME HEALTHCARE TELECOMMUNICATIONS PATHWAYS

Automated information systems encompass computerized databases and other software systems used in areas such as patient care, utilization review, quality assurance, education, cost accounting, and research. These tools are essential to shaping opportunities for improving and expanding healthcare to the home. The impetus for management information systems comes from the need for immediate retrieval of large volumes of data on provider productivity, appropriateness of services utilized, cost benefits, and outcomes of care. The quality of care depends on the accuracy of such information systems. These databases are essential to the evaluation of relative costs, resource utilization, and variations in service delivery. The fundamental information system is derived by building an electronic longitudinal patient record. Much like a credit reporting agency, the longitudinal patient record contains a comprehensive chronology of the individual's interaction with the healthcare system.

The Comprehensive Electronic Patient Record

The traditional paper trail of patient records is becoming digital. Trying to locate a patient's medical records, which are often lost in one of the many stages of processing, will increasingly become a thing of the past. The team approach to care management requires access to the patient's medical records on a 24-hour basis. The safety and care of patients may be seriously compromised in the absence of the electronic patient record.

Comprehensive practice management and computerized medical record systems that bring together audio, graphics, and video to create a fully integrated solution to billing and medical record problems of healthcare providers are now available.

Electronic Longitudinal Patient Record Systems

Electronic longitudinal patient record systems provide the following:

- Easy access to contextually sensitive knowledge and information for healthcare providers
- Accurate recording of clinical information
- Protocol-based treatment
- Outcome analysis
- Long-term follow-up

Because healthcare is an information-driven service, better care can be provided at less cost through computerized medical record systems that address the following concerns:

- Elimination of waste and decreased denial of reimbursement from erroneous claims submissions
- Avoidance of unnecessary and redundant test ordering
- Reduction in administrative and management overhead
- Knowledge bases that provide for appropriate resource utilization
- Accessing information about plan authorization requirements
- Managing and monitoring pharmaceuticals through controlled formularies
- Accessing information about laboratory tests and medications to facilitate informed decisions between patients and physicians
- Analyzing outcomes to improve delivery and the cost of care
- Patient education and empowerment programs to facilitate informed decisions
- Self-management

Dr. Mark L. Braunstein, President and CEO of Patient Care Technologies, Inc., claims that "a practical structured electronic record must be based upon a predefined, consistent nomenclature within an equally defined structure. Within such a system, each clinical concept (e.g., individual assessments, care plans, and interventions to use home care nursing terminology) can be thought of as a 'building block' upon which the chart is built. Within each concept are the detailed observations normally associated with the element of care. These building blocks become the foundation for critical pathways."[2]

Critical Pathways

Critical pathways are a set of guidelines that do the following:[2]

- Link the appropriate elements of care to each diagnosis/acuity level
- Provide a suggested approach for performing the care elements over time
- Lay out the appropriate goals for each segment of care and the appropriate measures of outcomes versus the goals
- Provide the basis for analysis of variation

Features to Consider

Features to consider when selecting a patient record system include the following:

Log-on Security
Customized data retrieval
System security

Registration Module
Patient demographics
Patient photo capture

Billing Module
CPT and ICD-9-CM coding
Claims submission
Line item entry
Automated physician referral letters
Billing forms
Integration with medical records module

Reporting Module
Managed care
Accounting
Graphing and charting
Custom

Pharmacy Module
Drug information
Drugs listed by category
Drug formulary
Patient medication list
Automated prescription writing

Medical Record Module

Listings of complete or incomplete medical records

Laboratory results with integration services

Integrated radiological reporting and radiograph viewing

Integrated digital dictation system

Support for digital cameras and scanners

Multimedia video support

Automated linking between diagnosis and plan selections with CPT coding and matching ICD-9-CM codes, including complete codes knowledge base

Customization to personal ICD-9-CM listing

Tailored medical record printout

Integrated transcriptions

Word processing

Patient diagnoses list

Graphics that transfer to medical record

Drawing and sketching

Cost breakdowns for all testing, supplies, drugs, services, and reimbursement rates

Protocol system (for both use and generation)

Dates of visits and corresponding medical records

Patient problem list with matching medical records

Printing and faxing of physician referral letters

On-line Information Networks

The Internet currently links diverse and distant people at levels never before anticipated, and its role in healthcare is expanding. Providers are rapidly building Web sites to inform, expose, and advertise healthcare products and services. Consumers are using the Internet to acquire information, explore, and buy healthcare products and services directly from their homes. While the accuracy of information on the Internet has been an issue, the number of credible Web sites sponsored by responsible organizations continues to grow.

Web sites already include nearly every healthcare topic imaginable. The World Wide Web is becoming the global network of choice for obtaining consumer information, and it will increasingly serve to educate and inform patients, who are now becoming more involved in the management of their own health problems. Web sites are evolving at a staggering rate, and they have information on local, regional, and national healthcare products and services, including support groups and chat rooms. Although the Internet will probably continue to be the largest single source of healthcare information, local and regional provider service networks will provide secure, targeted applications specific to the needs of patients at a much faster pace.

Community Health Information Networks (CHINs) and central on-line repositories for patient medical records are being established to create access to current and historical patient information and provide patient self-management features for the home healthcare industry. These networks can be regional or national, which enables electronic transactions, including claims billings to HCFA. Hand-held devices are now available so that home healthcare nurses can input all clinical information while at the patient's home and transfer it by modem to the local home healthcare agency or network using regular telephone lines.

Video and Television

Video and television are going through similar growth, particularly in regard to the emergence of digital and high-definition television (HDTV). Once the specifications have been agreed upon, the potential for applications in home healthcare will be immense. Currently, HHT applications are very limited because of the wiring requirements for interactive television. There is no doubt about the values of interactive television as a tool for treating homebound patients, particularly in regard to the psychosocial aspects of care. The main problem is the cost and time required to wire America for such technology.

Operational Problems and HHT Benefits

The American Medical Association (AMA) has gone on record to support the value of home healthcare in reducing patient and family stress caused by physical, emotional, and financial difficulties.[3] The benefits are attributed to the participation of the family in both planning and implementing the patient's treatment based on the outpatient examination. There is overwhelming evidence in support of the role of home healthcare in improving access, helping improve patient conditions in less time, and facilitating interventions earlier in the disease process. To support these initiatives, the AMA issued in 1998 a set of guidelines for physicians involved in telehealth.

One company that has been an innovator in telehealth is HELP Innovations, Inc. They have identified a number of potential opportunities for delivering telehealth services. Among them are:[4]

- Healthcare delivery in remote geographical areas
- Patients who are at risk for nursing home placement
- Patients who are at high-risk for complications
- Patients who receive a high volume of services or high-cost services
- Patients who are non-compliant with taking their medications
- Patients who have chronic diseases or conditions
- Patients who require special care

HELP Innovations' ResourceLink™ services relies on a strategy that is cost effective and uses viable communications. The company's goal is to meet patient needs in any geographical area while maintaining the flexibility to incorporate new technologies as they emerge. The media they currently use includes a mixture of the telephone, cable, and integrated services digital network (ISDN) technology applied in the most cost-effective manner while considering the inherent strengths and weaknesses of these technologies. There are many benefits to the ResourceLink strategy.[5]

Benefits of the ResourceLink strategy may include:

Benefits for the Patient

- Increased sense of control and independence with caregivers
- Ability to remain at home
- Quality care
- Ease of use
- More timely and convenient visits

- Improved compliance in taking medications

Benefits for the Home Healthcare Provider (Other than Homecare Agency)

- Enhancement of traditional home healthcare services
- Ability to educate the patient and family regarding disease management
- Enhanced ability to monitor the patient's health status
- Reduced travel and documentation time
- Ability to visualize and interact with the patient
- Easy to install and use

Benefits for the Physician

- Consistent monitoring of patient compliance
- Improved patient outcomes
- Immediate notification of changes in the patient's condition
- Printed reports of the patient's status

Benefits for the Home Healthcare Agency

- Reduced travel costs
- Increased productivity of nurses
- Increased range of services offered
- Visits delivered at less cost
- Increased quality control capabilities

SUPPORT SERVICES

Among the support services required for HHT applications are a combination of technological solutions and deliverable services. Interactive video with patient management software support offers quick and timely interactions and immediate interventions. Access to patient files on-line enables providers to make a single entry of patient information, reducing paperwork. Costs are reduced by decreasing the amount of travel to the patient's homes and by using existing telephone lines in the patient's home.

Technical Solutions

Strategies using the information superhighway that have been proposed by some industry leaders require further study. There is much focus on investments through entertainment services, although there are not significant data about the level of consumer interest in broadband applications, such as video-on-demand, gambling, interactive games, and home shopping.

Among certain communication industry executives, the underlying assumption is that if something is offered, the public will use it—a theory based on the history of the telephone, television, and video recorder. They could be right, and many people have concluded that it might just take more time for people to make such a shift.

Based on a national public-opinion survey of 600 adults, respondents indicated they wanted "on-line capabilities such as on-demand access to reference materials; educational courses or how-to programs that allow interaction with [the] class or instructor (distance learning); interactive reports on local schools; and access [to] information about government services and training."[6] The greatest number of respondents indicated they would be more willing to pay for such services.

It should be noted that various attempts at legislation designed to deregulate telecommunications and cable companies are ongoing. The rationale is that open competition will provide consumers with a greater diversity of choice. Ultimately, the convergence of key participants may be necessary to resolve the issues essential to making progress in establishing broadband interactive networks.

Deliverables

What will be deliverable services in the next few years? Underlying the task of developing large interactive networks is a growing effort to provide what people really want through ISDN and other high-speed technologies using existing telephone lines. Such an interactive solution could meet both the true needs of the public while establishing the market needed to finance broadband networks.

The balance of evidence suggests that a combination of HHT technologies will be in place, including broadband demonstration projects and the establishment of limited networks in heavily populated urban centers and isolated rural areas with support from the federal government by the year 2000.

Telephony manufacturers and vendors could take the lead in meeting many of the current needs in education and health while the long-range broadband effort is being integrated over the years ahead. Authorities predict it will be at least a decade before the logistical, technical, legal, political, and financial barriers will be resolved, clearing the way for the establishment of broadband networks.

The deliverable that will reach the greatest numbers in the shortest time and meet the most needs of consumers is telephony.

IMPORTANT CONSIDERATIONS AND QUESTIONS

Among the many important considerations and questions of telecommunications and home healthcare are cost and policy problems that require pathbuilding initiatives for their resolution.

Cost and Policy Issues

HHT cost and policy are inseparable factors in the shaping of the future of home healthcare. The true value of HHT must be systematically researched and demonstrated before any real progress can be made in resolving policy issues of cost benefits, access, infrastructure, and professional participation.

Cost Benefits and Access

Improved cost benefits and access have enabled the home healthcare industry to establish a foundation on which to build HHT applications. Researchers in healthcare substantiate the potential of HHT for expanding access, reducing costs, and improving the quality of healthcare. These observations have wide support in both the United States and Canada.

Among the many barriers that must be overcome is the need to improve access and increase use with less cost. Access to basic healthcare should be available for all people. The focus should be on the many benefits, including reducing the cost of providing home healthcare through the implementation of technology. The values of preventative care must also be included in the long-range formula for determining the human and financial benefits of HHT applications.

Cost issues evolve from the question of who is going to pay for the required telecommunications services needed to launch the research and to ultimately implement proven HHT applications. There is a growing consensus that the key to this question is partnering. Federal, state, and local governments must collaborate with industry in planning and financing the technological infrastructure.

Infrastructure

Developing the infrastructure through partnerships between government and industry is not a new concept. It was done in the establishment of national telephone networks, railways, and coast-to-coast highway and interstate systems. Currently, many states are collaborating with universities and private industry to establish demonstration projects using telecommunications networks that are capable of providing two-way interactive video. Indeed, this may be the beginning of HHT application expansion.

Given the revolution in information transfer created by the Internet, it is inevitable that the telecommunications superhighway will become the next major focus. This effort will be required by government in partnership with industry—revisiting a highly essential and successful approach from the past. Because the Internet is becoming overwhelmed by users and cannot meet the demands for service, the issue may be resolved by the voters themselves, provided that they become informed. This will require additional research to demonstrate the capacity of HHT to provide the kinds of healthcare services that are effective, affordable, and acceptable to both providers and patients.

Mary Gardner Jones of the Consumer Interest Research Institute claims "the Telecommunications Act of 1996 and the FCC's Universal Service Rules implementing the healthcare provisions of the Act have taken a conservative view of the potential of the national information infrastructure (NNI) to promote community and individual health."[7] The FCC is currently making a cautious start toward enabling rural communities to establish telecommunications networks to provide healthcare services to patients. This beginning will help to validate telemedicine as a viable resource and lay the foundation for the development of HHT applications.

Perhaps a strategy that addresses the needs of the community for education, economic development, government information, and human and health services is the correct formula for the partnerships required between industry and government to move forward. In any event, "until these advanced networks are universally deployed [in] the home, the absence of these networks will stand as the single most important barrier to patients' access in their homes to the full range of home [health]care services which are so essential to their well-being and to the development of a more cost-effective, high-quality healthcare system."[8]

The issue of cost is rapidly shifting focus from benefits to implementation, and this must be addressed by solutions that respond to politics, partnerships, and joint resources.

Professional Participation

Professional participation requires the removal of barriers in insurance coverage, reimbursement policies, licensure, confidentiality, and quality of information.[9]

Third-party insurance and Medicare provide limited home healthcare services following inpatient care, and vital contributions could be made in certain preventive applications, treatment of chronic illnesses, and support services. Medicaid, however, is a large source of support for home and community long-term healthcare. The Medicaid waiver program does partially fill this gap by providing home healthcare, medications, and transportation services for those in the low-income bracket.

There is strong evidence for major cost benefits (resulting from certain electronically delivered home healthcare services) beyond having a physician present at both ends of the communication pathway. HCFA is now beginning to acknowledge the role of home healthcare in provision of triage, emergency consultations, follow-up services after certain inpatient visits, and healthcare services for rural patients and underserved groups in metropolitan areas.

Providers must also have incentives to provide home healthcare. With existing HHT applications, reimbursement policies are easier to determine. HCFA must take a more proactive stance in identifying and reimbursing the most obvious cost-effective HHT applications, which could possibly provide the necessary incentive for the industry to respond by developing and implementing the technology required to deliver such services. The final solution for establishing the most cost-effective way to provide healthcare services to patients—wherever the location—absolutely must be reimbursed by both government and health insurance providers.

The provision of HHT applications is global and exceeds geographical boundaries, much like the Internet. State licensure restrictions are another barrier to the delivery of care, particularly in underserved rural areas, where appropriate professional healthcare providers could deliver much-needed services. With the advent of HHT applications, state licensing bodies should develop reciprocity policies or cooperative licensure mechanisms to provide the most appropriate type of caregiver for those in need.

Maintaining confidentiality of patient records, which are fundamentally the property of the patient, and providing reliable care delivery are absolutes that must be considered when preparing for HHT applications. The patient's identity must be kept private and protected from intruders. Providers must be willing to share and use electronic healthcare records through network systems. The issue of whether to expose one's treatment plans and medical decisions provides another potential barrier among physicians.

Pathbuilding Initiatives

In the Consumer Interest Research Institute report Electronic House Calls: 21st Century Options, Mary Gardner Jones provided the following proposed recommendations for future steps to promote the electronic delivery of home healthcare:[10]

1. Development of a national long-term care policy which supports and provides for the delivery of a continuum of medical and social services in a continuum of facilities must encompass the following components:

   - State and federal reform and support for healthcare services that maximizes achievable outcomes and independence by patients in their homes
   - Reimbursement policies that support long-term care whenever possible within home
   - Development of quality standards for all provider institutions, including appropriate training and competency standards for care delivery and supervision of care providers and care takers, including appropriate licensure and certification systems, and consumer grievance procedures open for public inspection
   - Establishment of compensation and benefits for long-term care providers in the home that recognizes skills, responsibility, quality of care, and availability of personnel

2. Timely deployment of advanced telecommunications networks to the home must be implemented on both the national and local levels through the following steps:

   - Promote adoption of a long-range national telecommunications goal by the federal government to create universal service capable of delivering and receiving affordable and accessible high-quality audio, video, data, and graphics by users
   - Create incentives for the appropriate market that will promote the universal deployment of advanced telecommunications network links to the home
   - Create partnerships between appropriate government agencies, industry, and coalitions to

develop and implement a strategic plan to establish these network applications

3. Revision of current healthcare reimbursement and licensure regulations affecting home care through the following steps:

 - Adoption by HCFA of the recommendations of the Center For Health Policy Research and extension of the recommended initial coverage to persons receiving electronically delivered long-term home care services without which these patients would require institutionalization.

 - Revision of current HCFA reimbursement policies to ensure that home care services are covered whether provided in person or through HHT, when appropriate; [that] coverage of services and medications do not discriminate against the provision of home care; [and that] coverage of all licensed healthcare professionals providing home care services [are] in accordance with a physician approved plan of care

 - Re-examination of state licensure laws to ensure that reasonable and timely home healthcare will not be denied due to a lack of local manpower resources, local disasters, or state boundaries

 - Development of standards of transmission resolution requirements for the delivery of various healthcare services to ensure quality of care

 - National enactment of a comprehensive privacy statute that prohibits the sale or lease of personally identified patient healthcare data, inappropriate disclosure, and standards for disclosure for healthcare purposes

4. Promotion of quality of healthcare information, designed with privacy safeguards and assurances of provider cooperation in electronic healthcare information and record systems by ensuring [the following]:

- Appropriate terms and conditions will be agreed upon by care providers and consumers as to the use of patient record data.
- Community health information networks are designed to capture patients' healthcare services delivered in their homes and contain effective privacy and security safeguards.
- Development of common languages and standards to facilitate consumer access to health information, and tools to cope with information problems.

5. Creation of citizen and healthcare professional educational outreach programs by encouraging:
- Local groups, institutions, and consumer organizations to establish coalitions with healthcare and educational professionals and industry to inform and educate the public as to the home health benefits of advanced telecommunications networks and the role of government in making these benefits possible
- Media and educational campaigns to promote the use of HHT
- Provider organizations and providers to develop training programs in the use of HHT
- Development by professional medical associations of comprehensive programs to inform and educate their members as to the medical and cost benefits of HHT
- Medical schools to develop clinical telemedicine programs to prepare students to use HHT applications in rural and medically underserved communities

6. Promotion of research studies on electronically delivered home care designed to:
- Document comparative costs and medical effects of home healthcare for all possible and appropriate applications

- Analyze the value and cost effectiveness of delivering heath care services electronically to patients' homes
- Determine the impact of HHT applications on different population groups and on the healthcare system in general on the equity of access and quality of care[11]

For a complete description of these pathbuilding initiatives, the reader should refer to the original document by the Consumer Interest Research Institute.

CONCLUSION

The merger of telecommunications and healthcare requires pathbuilding initiatives that facilitate HHT applications. The initiatives involve policy issues and the deployment of advanced telecommunications networks in the home. Important factors of the process are the revision of reimbursement and licensure regulations, promotion of quality health information, educational outreach programs, and research. The marriage of these industries can only be consummated by merging the science and culture of telecommunications technology with medicine and healthcare delivery.

REFERENCES

1. Mary Gardner Jones, *Electronic House Calls: 21st Century Options*, June 1995, Consumer Interest Research Institute.
2. Personal communication with Mark L. Braunstein, President and CEO of Patient Care Technologies, Inc., October 29, 1998.
3. E. Andrew Balls, Farad J., Gilad J.K., et al.: Electronic Communication With Parents: Evaluation of Distance Medicine Technology, *JAMA* 278(no. 2), 1997, pp. 152–159.
4. Linda L. Roman: *ResourceLink™*, HELP Innovations, Lawrence, KS, 1997.
5. Ibid.
6. Charles Piller: Dreamnet, *Macworld,* October 1994, p. 99.
7. Jones op. cit.
8. Ibid.
9. Ibid.
10. Ibid.
11. Ibid.

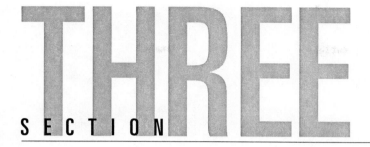

BEYOND THE YEAR 2000

7

CHAPTER

Future Challenges

In her writing as early as 1900, Florence Nightingale used the term *home nursing* in the same sense as it is used today. She discussed patient's homes as the setting where nursing care should be provided. She said, "Nursing care provided to individuals in their own homes is more desirable and could replace hospitalization, because in their homes patients could be helped to feel the independence of their life."[1]

OVERVIEW

This chapter discusses future challenges as they relate to healthcare providers, manufacturers, and suppliers with interests specific to home healthcare. Strategies are explored that offer suggestions for responding to future challenges and assisting in creating opportunities.

Areas addressed in this chapter are:

- An industry analysis
- A closer look at factors driving the industry
- Strategies for change

INDUSTRY ANALYSIS

The healthcare industry is one of the fastest growing industries both in the U.S. and throughout the world. Along with this growth comes rapid change as the industry of healthcare begins to transform itself and adopt standard business practices in an effort to keep current with the changes and compete in a demanding environment. These practices are mostly aimed at improving efficiencies and reducing costs.

Navigating the maze of regulatory and reimbursement challenges will require focused leadership with a clear vision. In the changing world of healthcare, flexible and dynamic management will usher in success, whereas complacency will cause failure. This fluid state produces a type of natural selection in the evolution of business that often results in new and different archetypes. Charles Darwin stated, "It is not the strongest of the species that survive, nor the most intelligent, but the most responsive to change."

These new models and different methodologies are already beginning to emerge as this new order of natural selection takes hold in the healthcare industry. New technologies, the obsolescence of entitlements, economics, and changing demographics will all contribute to the way in which healthcare services are delivered in the future.

The U.S. spent almost $1.1 trillion on healthcare in 1997. Yet both proprietary and not-for-profit hospital systems report filling just over half of their beds. In addition, they have experienced shortened lengths of stays. This supports the idea that the healthcare industry is aggressively pursuing less costly avenues for providing care.

As government and managed care payers continue to affect the industry, there is a trend toward moving patients from acute care hospitals to other settings. It is becoming more common for patients to be transferred earlier to nursing homes or to their own residences, where they receive care through home healthcare agencies. As hospitals and other institutional providers experience a decrease in utilization, some of these facilities will shift their beds to other services.[2]

Factors Driving the Industry

The healthcare industry is in an evolutionary stage. Although it is important to view an industry in terms of its growth stage, it is also critical to determine the causes for the change.

The most dominant forces that create the impetus for change are called driving forces. These driving forces will have a great influence on the types of changes that will occur in an industry.[3]

There are various elements that are precipitating changes in the healthcare industry. They include:

1. The economic climate: changes in regulatory and reimbursement methodologies, including managed care
2. Incidence and prevalence of patient condition
3. Research and development, advances in technology
4. Demographics

THE ECONOMIC CLIMATE: CHANGES IN REGULATORY AND REIMBURSEMENT METHODOLOGIES

Until the advent of managed care and the Health Care Finance Administration (HCFA) enacted OBRA in 1987, there were few systematic approaches to healthcare reimbursement. Basically, when someone became ill, his or her physician would admit him or her to the hospital. Treatment continued until the patient recovered, with little regard to length of stay. The insurance plan was billed, and the patient made arrangements to pay the deductible. Insurance plans passed along their increases by raising the premiums. The taxpayer paid the price for those in the Medicaid and Medicare systems, and the employer bore the burden for the employee's health insurance premiums.

MEDICARE

In the late 1980s, everything changed. HCFA enacted the Omnibus Budget Reconciliation Act, more commonly known as OBRA. This act designated criteria that regulated how providers were paid. Further it introduced limits on lengths of stays directly related to type and severity of diagnosis.

Patients were now being discharged after a shortened hospital stay, and acute care facilities were scrambling to find appropriate settings for disposition. This impacted greatly on the development and expansion of post-acute care. Growth could be observed in the areas of skilled nursing facilities, specialty programs, outpatient clinics, ambulatory care sites, and home healthcare.

In 1997 the U.S. Congress passed the Balanced Budget Act (BBA), and with it came sweeping reforms in healthcare regulations and reimbursement. This Act will be implemented over a period of years. One of the new reforms which impacts most healthcare providers is the Prospective Payment System (PPS).

The PPS once again cuts into the revenue streams of the providers and affects virtually every aspect of the healthcare industry that offers care to Medicare recipients. As an example, the rates of payment for home healthcare services will in many cases be reduced. This will cause a trickle-down effect that impacts every supplier, manufacturer, and vendor to the industry.

It has been suggested that profit margins may shrink as much as 25% in what is already a beleaguered industry. Essentially PPS will make OBRA look like a walk in the park to many providers. This might explain the new flurry of consolidations among healthcare providers.

PPS will also require that providers supply specific information, in a certain format, under strict time constraints. This means the use of electronic data transfer that necessitates computers, special programs, software, and telecommunications. Although some of these elements may already be in place at some organizations, unfortunately this is not the standard. Even those who do employ these mechanisms understand that the rules have changed and that there will be a significant learning curve over the next decade.

All of this would not be worth mentioning if the Medicare population were insignificant; however, just the opposite is true. The elderly population, which represents the majority of Medicare patients, is expanding rapidly. The aging process often makes people more vulnerable to illnesses that might require medical intervention.

The growth of after-hospital or post-acute care and other than hospital or alternate-site care, is directly proportional to the increase in Medicare beneficiaries. HCFA estimates that there were 39 million people enrolled in the Medicare program in 1997. In that same year, 10% of these beneficiaries were purchasers of home healthcare services (twice the number of purchasers since 1990).

In addition to the new reimbursement rules, HCFA is taking a tougher stance on fraud and abuse of the financial system. A new provision called Operation Restore Trust (ORT) to monitor activities has been introduced, and beneficiaries are even being recruited to assist in the compliance effort.

MANAGED CARE

History will reveal that one of the most important drivers of change in the healthcare industry, in the last decades of the 20th century, was the development of managed care. Increases in costs and growth in the size of the healthcare industry led to the implementation of managed care.

The term managed care has come to be used interchangeably with health maintenance organizations more commonly known as HMOs. It is important to note that HMOs are not the only form of managed care.

In fact, there are many models of managed care systems and services, including preferred provider organizations or PPOs. Although many managed care organizations have varied system methods, they all operate under the premise that, in return for delivering a significant volume of business, providers agree to offer services to managed care members at a pre-negotiated price, and often within structured guidelines.

Managed care enrollment reached approximately 60 million members and their families in 1997. This critical mass in highly penetrated markets is forcing greater competition. These payers are tough negotiators and demanding buyers as they must live up to their promise of making healthcare services available at fixed costs.

There are various ways in which managed care organizations structure reimbursement. The following represent the
most common types:

- **Discounted fee-for-service**—Usually represented by
  a percentage off the usual and customary charges,
  considered to be the least risky method for the provider
- **Pre-negotiated rates**—Based on treatments or
  services offered, this takes the form of per-diem, per-
  visit or per procedure rates, and extends a small
  amount of risk for the provider
- **Capitated rates**—Demonstrated by both the payer and
  the provider sharing risk; often implemented on a per-
  member/per-month basis or a percentage thereof
- **Case rates**—A prescribed rate for caring for a patient
  with a specific incident or diagnosis for the life of that
  occurrence. For instance, a hospital may have a
  case-rate contract for persons who are admitted with a
  diagnosis of appendicitis, and the case rate would
  require that the hospital provide appropriate care for
  the duration of the patient's appendicitis including any
  surgery, medications, and or treatments necessary. The
  case rate, obviously, represents the greatest risk to the
  provider.

Managed care companies can factor into their budget pre-
determined rates, such as those that are capitated. The consideration that will drive this type of pricing is volume, by way of
employers as they increase their awareness of the cost savings
of managed care, and by those persons who receive government
reimbursement for their care, such as Medicare and Medicaid
recipients.

Managed care for public and private organizations is viewed
as an attractive alternative for reducing costs, both directly and
indirectly. A Price Waterhouse study conducted in 1995 showed
HMOs to be effective for employers and government recipients
by controlling the costs of their own beneficiaries more efficiently
and decreasing healthcare expenditures by impacting practice
patterns of professional and institutional providers.

The study indicated that for every 10% increase in penetration for a given market of Medicare Managed Care HMO or Medicare Risk HMO, as they are often referred to, the fee-for-service segment costs drop by almost 8%. This has vast implications for the Federal Budget, especially as the elderly population continues to expand (Figure 7–1).

This system will become more popular as more Medicare and Medicaid beneficiaries enroll in managed care plans. The potential dollars that this population represents is staggering.

In 1996, 16% of the 39 million Medicare beneficiaries were already enrolled in HMOs. The Western Regions led all other regions in both Medicare-Managed-Care and Medicaid-Managed-Care penetration. California had the largest percentage of Medicare Managed Care enrollees.

FIGURE 7–1

Estimated Annual Savings as Penetration Increases for Medicare Risk HMOs

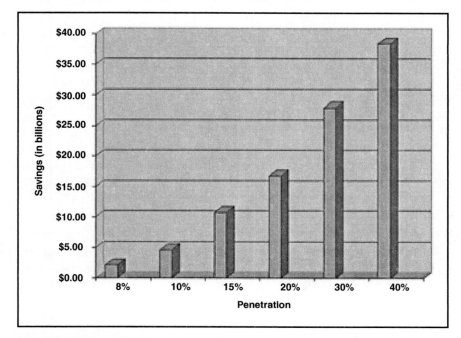

Source: PriceWaterhouse, 1995.

THE GLOBAL HEALTH ECONOMY

It is naive to speak of healthcare issues without mention of a global perspective. Financial situations in other countries are shifting, and they impact each other through a global marketplace. When stock markets in other nations, for example Japan, rise or fall, the sound of the closing bell is heard around the world.

The healthcare industry is now, more than ever, a part of this global market. This translates into big business. Pharmaceutical companies now mass-produce medications in plants around the world. Manufacturers of durable medical equipment, such as specialty beds, respiratory supplies, and wheelchairs, have factories located in many foreign countries. Suppliers and large distributors of these goods are engaged in worldwide delivery systems.

Some publicly traded corporations have enjoyed enormous profits over the past few years due to strong economies in developed countries throughout a global marketplace. Much of the relocation of healthcare manufacturers has been a response to shrinking reimbursement in countries such as the U.S. It is in the best interests of a corporation and its stockholders to trim costs in order to maintain profit margins.

Another element is ease of travel. It wasn't too many years ago, that even air travel was time-consuming, costly, and usually reserved only for the rich. Today, it is not only readily available, it is also a matter of course for most organizations engaged in international trade. Worldwide travel can be a double-edged sword. It allows freedom of movement for persons traveling between countries; however, it also provides for transportation of organisms such as bacteria and viruses. The introduction of new organisms and diseases can have disastrous results, as was recently witnessed with Ebola, HIV, and new strains of Tuberculosis. Some public health officials have predicted that, in the future, we will be fighting a worldwide war against communicable diseases that are yet unknown.

A factor encouraging the global marketplace, is the emergence of the information age. Never before has it been so expedient to communicate, create networks, and share information on a worldwide scale. New technologies are making it easier to produce, market, and distribute products globally while decreasing the costs of operation. Healthcare providers should expect to benefit from some of these cost savings.

Also, many countries around the world are experiencing changes in demographics—much like the United States, including growth in their elderly populations. Many countries such as Canada, Australia, the Scandinavian Countries, Japan, China, England, and Germany are studying the U.S. system of healthcare. These and other nations find their economies burdened by healthcare costs, and as a result, are developing many of the more recent U.S. healthcare models, such as alternate site care, work recovery programs, rehabilitation, case management, employer-sponsored risk assessment programs, and managed care. It is likely that the future leaders of nations will look to promote more collaborative efforts in healthcare.

INCIDENCE AND PREVALENCE OF DISEASE

The population trends, in combination with travel and the introduction of new and or resistant strains of bacteria are the winds of change swirling around the world's ability to combat illnesses. These are the issues that are making the 6 o'clock news and will become more prominent in the third millennium.

However, there are more familiar diseases in the eye of the storm. For instance, cardiac disease still claims the number one position of the top ten causes of death in the U.S. This data was published in the 1997 issue of the "Monthly Vital Statistics Report," by the National Center for Health Statistics and Healthy People 2000 from the U.S. Department of Health and Human Services (Figure 7–2).

Although science has made great strides in medicine, these statistics are an indication that there is still much to be done. The U.S. is in the forefront of healthcare innovation and technology, and will no doubt, continue to make new discoveries at a rapid rate.

FIGURE 7–2

Top Ten Causes of Death in the U.S.

Cause of Death	Deaths in 1995	Associated Risks
1. Heart disease	737,563	Lack of exercise Cholesterol Diet Diabetes High blood pressure Tobacco use Stress
2. Cancer	538,455	Diet Tobacco use Lack of check-ups Radon exposure
3. Cerebrovascular disease	157,991	(See heart disease risks)
4. Lung disease	102,899	Exercise Smoking
5. Accidental injury and adverse effects	93,320	Alcohol use Lack of injury control Seat belts Smoke detectors
6. Pneumonia and influenza	82,923	Smoking Other complications
7. Diabetes mellitus	59,254	Diet Exercise Weight
8. Acquired immune deficiency syndrome (AIDS)	43,115	Unprotected sex IV drug use
9. Suicide	31,284	Stress Firearms use
10. Liver disease and cirrhosis	25,222	Alcohol use

Source: National Center for Health Statistics, 1997.

RESEARCH AND DEVELOPMENT

The last century has seen prodigious gains in healthcare technologies and treatments. Technology has had a hand in advancing every aspect of healthcare, including how professionals communicate their findings. Computers, telecommunications, satellites, and the development of the integrated services digital network (ISDN) will serve as a foundation upon which we will build a new century of opportunities.

Some of these discoveries have led to such technologies that enable minimally invasive surgeries to be performed. New surgical instruments that are less invasive are making it possible for surgeons to guide procedures using videos and robotics. Fiber optic cable, dissolving sutures, microscopic techniques, and lasers have all made their way into the surgical suites of hospitals, spawning an industry of outpatient or ambulatory surgery centers.

Recent imaging apparatus and other new technologies offer a host of diagnostic equipment. These techniques are providing an alternative to invasive exploratory procedures that only a few years ago, were in some cases, the only way to diagnose a problem. Today, modern diagnostic technologies allow discovery and solutions through external methods. This means earlier and more accurate diagnoses, and a better chance for recovery that can result in decreased costs.

Pharmaco-informatics allow researchers to simulate the synthesis of various combinations of chemical compounds. These sophisticated computer programs contribute to a reduction in time and therefore, costs of development of new drugs and treatment modalities.

Biotechnology, genetic discoveries, and pharmaceutical developments are advancing new therapies for illnesses that were once thought to be untreatable. The Human Genome Project is scheduled for completion in the beginning of the third millennium. This project will, in the end, map thousands of genetic strands within DNA. It is expected that this will create the navigational tool for scientists to treat maybe as many as 10,000 diseases that are thought to be genetically based, including some forms of cancer.

Telemedicine is now common verbiage among healthcare professionals. This has opened up numerous avenues of information sharing. For example, much has been reported about rural hospital physicians now having real-time access to urban physicians and university medical centers to assist them in providing treatment without delay or transporting patients over long distances.

Integrated Services Digital Network (ISDN) uses telephone technology and computers to send data and images. This will advance the ability to provide rapid, cost-effective information. Other new communication technologies, such as fiber optics, Asynchronous Transfer Mode (ATM), and frame relay, offer powerful advantages for the rapid flow of high-bandwidth information.

The Internet phone and the screen phone will bring technology into the home and will offer the consumer information to better manage their health needs. It also allows professionals greater access to monitor and respond to the complications often associated with chronic illness.

The U.S. Department of Defense is reviewing the use of video phone technology and data transport for disease management of some of its employees. The system will utilize call-center technology to monitor patient progress.

All of these scientific and technological advances make it possible to shift care from the hospital or other institutional settings to the home. This trend is expected to experience continued growth as it is both effective and efficient.

DEMOGRAPHICS

The over-65 population is one of the most rapidly growing segments in the U.S. It is estimated that by the year 2010, this group will be almost 30% greater than it was in 1990. Further, those above the age of 85 years old are expected to increase 100% between 1990 and 2010 (Figure 7–3).

The average life span in 1900 was 45 years for men and 47 years for women. Recently, that same time period has almost doubled as the average life span is approaching 80 years and rising. Currently, the American Association of Retired Persons (AARP) represents over 20% of the voters. Today, there are more U.S. citizens over the age of 65 years old than the entire population of Canada.

Barring any catastrophes, there appears to be no end in sight as the "baby boom" generation enters this category. This

FIGURE 7–3

Growth in Age 65+ Population

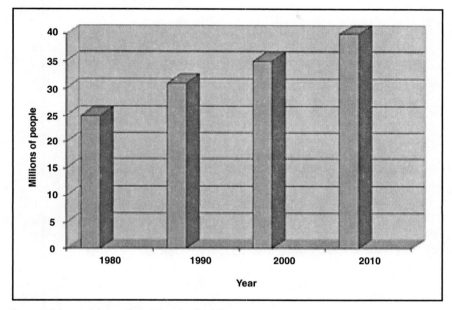

Source: U.S. Bureau of Census, Current Report on Population.

group is 76 million strong, and is a very powerful market. Here
are some examples that illustrate this point:

- Births climbed from under 3 million in 1946 to 4 million in
  1954 and then stayed at 4 million for 11 straight years.
- Revenues increased from products directed toward
  children, such as diapers and paper products.
- In 1940 less than 300 million jars of baby food were sold
  compared with 1.5 billion by 1954.
- The suburbs became the prized place to own a home.
- In 1957, there were more elementary schools built than
  ever before.
- As many boomers reached their teens, in 1967, more high
  schools were built then any other time in history.

- The teenager consumer spent $12 billion In 1964. Their parents spent another $13 billion on them.
- From 1965 to 1975 college enrollment almost tripled, going from 3.2 million to 9 million.
- In the 1970s, the boomers flooded the job market.
- In the 1980s, they created a baby boom of their own, topping 4 million births in 1989, a number which had only been achieved by their parents.
- In the 1990s, they became both the largest suppliers and purchasers of goods in the U.S.

This formidable group experienced nuclear testing, Dr. Spock, Mr. Spock, the Cold war, the Vietnam war, the Civil Rights war, the man on the moon, the Moonies, Moon Zappa, the hostage crisis, the war in Grenada, the Persian Gulf war, the war between the sexes, The Jonestown massacre, Mother Jones, keeping up with the Joneses, Nixon's "Checkers" speech, Nixon's checkered past, deflation, inflation, stagflation, Agent Orange, talent agents, the stock market's decline, the stock market's meteoric rise, earthquakes, hurricanes, tornadoes, floods, fires, mudslides, assassinations, inventions, art, color TV, FM radio, the microchip, the computer, the copy machine, the Internet, cloning, the de-industrialization of America, recession, mergers, acquisitions, takeovers, junk bonds, barges hauling junk, the trade deficit, rock and roll, rock slides, the Hard Rock Café, Watergate, Koreagate, Irangate, the collapse of the Berlin Wall, the collapse of the Soviet Union, riots, draughts, Woodstock, old age, the New Age, the information age, and Mother Theresa.

Through it all the baby boomers have demanded and created access to information. They will continue to be the "champions of change," affecting nearly every industry. The healthcare industry is no exception. As this group ages, they will by nature change the way healthcare is delivered in the U.S. as well as globally. One of the impacts is expected to be in the area of home healthcare and ambulatory care. Those providers of services with vision are already conducting research that will assist their organizations to plan for this customer base (Figures 7–4 and 7–5).

FIGURE 7–4

More Aches and Pains

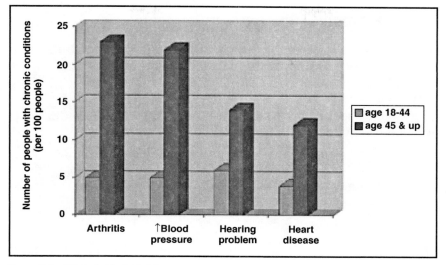

Source: National Center for Health Statistics.

FIGURE 7–5

Crises Multiply

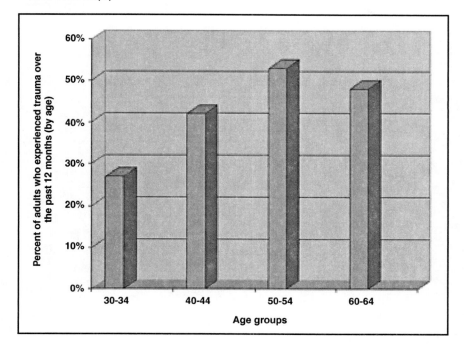

FUTURE STRATEGY AND INDUSTRY ANALYSIS

It is paramount in any industry to develop and sustain performance. If the healthcare industry is to maintain financial integrity without compromising quality, it will require leadership with a clear vision and a thoughtful strategy.

Five elements that determine the ability of any industry to achieve its goals are:

1. Ease of entry for competitors
2. Threat of substitutes
3. Buyers' leverage
4. Suppliers' leverage
5. Dynamics of competition[4]

The following chart may prove helpful as an overview (Figure 7–6).

FIGURE 7–6

Competitive Forces in High-Tech HHT

Ease of Competitor Entry	⟶	Difficult
Threat of Substitutes	⟶	Low to Moderate
Buyers' Leverage	⟶	Increasing
Suppliers' Leverage	⟶	Low
Dynamics of Competition	⟶	High

Ease of Competitor Entry

Healthcare, on some levels, is a community business. There was a time when consumers were willing to travel to receive specialty care, but now most people expect to receive care in their own town. In other words, even if you are a hospital or a home care provider that is part of a large corporation, it is still important to integrate into the community where you are geographically located.

With the advent of managed care and progress in technologies and treatments, hospital lengths of stays have decreased and there is greater non-hospital capability, such as home healthcare, skilled nursing facilities, assisted living, ambulatory care and outpatient centers.

This coupled with the efforts of industry leaders to establish a presence in major and minor markets, would make it difficult for new competitors to enter the marketplace. There are other barriers including the tremendous amount of start-up capital necessary; the difficult and often confusing licensing and regulatory requirements; and possible market saturation.

Of course, having said that, there are some opportunities in markets where a "carve out" or niche service is needed. This would however, require careful consideration and feasibility studies.

Threat of Substitutes

The threat of substitutes for home healthcare is low to moderate. These substitutes would take the form of ambulatory care sites that may engage in offering some similar services that are currently provided by home care agencies.

Some of these ambulatory care sites might include outpatient clinics that may offer rehabilitation therapy, or centers that provide respiratory or wound care and physician groups. The physician groups are those that have a large enough practice to make it financially feasible to have, for example, an infusion clinic.

The other factors that could influence substitution of home healthcare will be future discoveries in treatment methods, customer satisfaction and perception of choice of treatment site, and the attitudes of the purchasers.

Currently, home healthcare is considered to be one of the sites of choice to receive care. In addition, going to a physician office or ambulatory care clinic routinely, would require a certain level of mobility and function, as well as access to transportation. Many of the patients receiving home healthcare services are too ill or are non-ambulatory.

Buyers' Leverage

Buyers' leverage over healthcare providers is very high. Throughout the 1990s, managed care plans have experienced extraordinary growth. The number of enrollees dictates the amount of buying power that these plans maintain.

The aging population and the baby boom demographic will only perpetuate this growth if the current system remains relatively intact. As was mentioned previously, associations such as AARP and government agencies are encouraging their constituents to become managed care members.

Another faction that has enormous influence is America's employers. Most large employers offer healthcare insurance for their full-time workers, and these employers are unhappy with the rising costs. Many of these employers have recently or will undergo reorganization and or right-sizing and are looking for ways to cut down costs. Although employers have not yet exercised their buying muscle when it comes to health insurance, it is expected to be the next wave in precipitating change in healthcare services.

This purchasing power, albeit very high, is also considered to be a positive for home healthcare providers who offer high-tech services at lower costs than hospitals.

Suppliers' Leverage

Suppliers, in this case, represent those who provide goods and services to the industry, more specifically the home healthcare industry. At the present time, they are considered to have decreasing leverage. The exception to this would be a manufacturer or supplier of a one-of-a-kind product that is in great demand.

The new squeeze on reimbursement to the healthcare provider also has an effect on those who supply the industry. Managed care, large employers, and new government regulations, such as PPS, are forcing the provider to find alternative methods of controlling costs. This translates to all organizations that distribute to or make products for the home healthcare industry.

Essentially, fewer unnecessary tests are being ordered, generic drugs are being used almost exclusively, and manufacturers and vendors are being asked to be better business partners in an effort to help providers trim costs.

The information and technology industries are expected to lower the price of healthcare delivery even further by developing tools to increase the efficiencies of professional personnel. The visionary home healthcare provider will employ these tools to better position themselves to meet the challenges of the future.

Dynamics of Competition

Healthcare is a community business. The competitive environment and market characteristics are specific to each community. Home healthcare in most metropolitan areas is extremely competitive.

There are various issues that factor into this competitive environment, including the following:

1. Managed care penetration levels
2. Size of the market
3. Type and number of competitors
4. Demographics
5. Government payers
6. Employers

Payers

All of these components will impact the competitive market of a home healthcare provider. Managed care penetration levels, government payers and large employer groups will drive pricing in most markets. The rates that are negotiated will depend on the providers' ability to offer services at reduced costs, communicate data, track outcomes, and maintain quality and patient satisfaction.

As much of the reimbursement today is negotiated as all-inclusive rates or capitated payment, it is critical that the home healthcare provider form relationships with suppliers that foster profitability. These affiliations must involve all those who impact the home healthcare agency's ability to conduct business while maintaining strong financial integrity.

Market Size and Demographics

Size of the market and demographics go hand-in-hand. If the home healthcare agency is one of only a few that is located in an area that is highly populated; with low unemployment rates; and a substantial amount of elderly persons, then the chances of acquiring and maintaining growth are good.

However, if the same set of circumstances apply without the elderly population, it may not matter what the size of the market is because not enough people will require those services. Another consideration is the income of the clientele. Healthcare is no different from any other industry in that it exists on the ability of its customers to pay for the products or services rendered. There appears to be a direct correlation between age and affluence (Figure 7–7).

FIGURE 7–7

Affluence Hits Its Peak

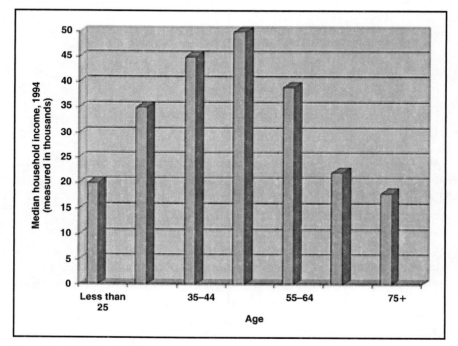

Source: National Center for Health Statistics, 1994.

It is just as important for the provider to carefully consider population and demographics in terms of payer mix. Most healthcare providers accept many types of reimbursement to maintain volume and cash-flow; however, they may have prepared their pro-forma financial statements based on specific levels of reimbursement.

The technology of today allows the home healthcare manager greater flexibility and knowledge about future budgetary projections through the use of simulated financial scenarios. A sophisticated program that can tie costs to charges and payments is a wise investment. Taking that concept one step further, there are programs and systems available now that provide that information and, in addition, integrate outcome data as a function of the total costs of care.

New technologies will also provide a vehicle to access a larger number of patients. The ability to track and monitor patients without having to hire more staff will allow the provider to increase revenues while incurring limited costs.

Type and Number of Competitors

With all of the regulations surrounding the healthcare industry, one would expect more definition, and yet the industry has been plagued by such rapid change that there is often a blurring of lines. One example of this is rehabilitation. When asked where rehabilitation therapy is provided, the answer may be, everywhere. There are, of course, some boundaries. Currently, acute inpatient rehabilitation requires that the patient be able to tolerate three hours of therapy a day. However, an outpatient or a home healthcare patient might also be able to tolerate three hours of therapy a day.

The clouding of these and other issues leave the provider community open to suspicion and further regulations. It confuses the consumer and the payer alike. On a positive note, an industry in a state of change also is open to new directions and opportunities.

Current competitors in home healthcare consist of:

- **High-tech home health organizations**—Usually medium to large organizations having many operations, spanning a regional to national area, with the ability to provide the full gamut of home care including those highly technical services.

- **Fully integrated healthcare systems**—The corporations both for-profit and not-for-profit comprising acute hospital(s), ambulatory and outpatient centers, and post-acute care programs that include skilled nursing facilities and home healthcare. The phrase "cradle to grave" is often applied.

- **Post-acute care continuums**—Similar to the concept of the fully integrated systems, but with a focus on other than hospital or alternate site care, usually skilled nursing facility(s), assisted living, adult day care, home healthcare, and various ancillary services, such as rehabilitation therapy and pharmacy.

- **Physician groups**—Most of their entry into the home healthcare arena consists of large medical groups providing some aspect of home healthcare services, such as infusion clinics.

- **Ambulatory care centers**—Competition with home healthcare mostly in their ability to offer service(s) to those patients who are somewhat mobile and have access to transportation.

- **Freestanding home healthcare agencies**—Smaller organizations that may have many of the capabilities of the large home healthcare organizations, but lack the network and the purchasing power.

- **Low-tech home healthcare**—Generally these are the agencies that provide caregivers to those who require some assistance with activities of daily living (ADLs). They often include personal aids, housekeepers, someone to help with shopping or to pay bills. They provide a necessary and growing service.

All of the organizations listed are part of a large field of competitors in the home healthcare industry (Figure 7–8). While some are vying for a similar client base, all of these providers represent competition as reimbursement continues to decrease and they contend for market share.

FIGURE 7-8

Strategic Group Map

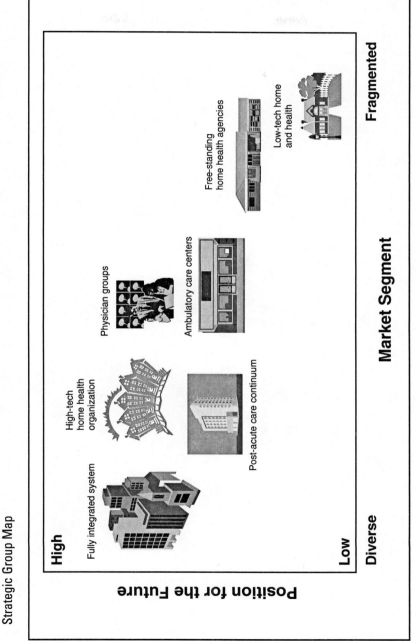

REFERENCES

1. Florence Nightingale's Concept of Home Nursing, *Japanese Journal of Nursing Research*, 1997.

2. Roussel: *Managed Care Digest Series* p. 40, Kansas City, 1997, SMG Marketing Group Inc.

3. A. Thompson, Strickland, A.: *Crafting and Implementing Strategy*, p. 85, New York, 1998, McGraw-Hill.

4. Michael E. Porter: *Competitive Strategy*, p. 142, New York, 1980, Simon & Schuster.

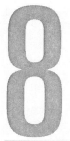

CHAPTER

The Age of Information Transfer

Imagining the future of home healthcare begins with a healthy respect for history as well as current demographic and social trends. The future vision grows based on the potential power of telecommunications and technology, and crests with an optimistic belief that structural inefficiency, given enough time, will be righted by well-meaning and informed people. One projection for the future comprises the interlocking of transformational processes and outcomes that may define a different home healthcare world than we know today.

The purpose of this chapter is to underscore the importance of information transfer (IT). We will also chance a glimpse into the future to project how technology might affect healthcare, and particularly homecare.

WHAT GOES AROUND, COMES AROUND

In the early 1800s, Americans received their healthcare at home. Doctors made house calls and brought everything they needed for diagnosis and treatment with them. What they lacked in high-powered instrumentation, they made up for in their powers of observation and concern for their patients. The family doctor was a tower of respect in a rough and tumble society, and patients who failed to comply with his orders did so at their own medical and social peril.

Sick people liked being treated at home. It was convenient, and they were in familiar surroundings during a stressful time. Their loved ones were nearby to assist them in getting better, and these caregivers played a pivotal role in the treatment plan.

Things began to change, however, by the early 1900s. The advent of cars and telephones, and a growing middle class made hospitalization more feasible and accessible. Important medical developments, such as x-rays, aseptic surgical practices, professional nursing, and physician licensing were reflected as improvements in care. As hospitals became better organized and had better equipment, they began to provide specialized care using tools that couldn't be transported easily to the home. Consequently, healthcare professionals left people's homes and relocated to the nation's growing number of hospitals.

This shift from the home to the hospital intensified during the 20th century. By 1980, there were more than 7,500 hospitals around the country. Yet, for reasons detailed earlier in this book, the pendulum is swinging back. At the turn of the century, we will see that there are fewer than 6,000 hospitals in the U.S. In another two decades, there may be half that number. At the same time, home healthcare is where the action is—growing faster than any other segment of healthcare, and faster than just about every other industry.

As "baby boomers" and their parents get older, the demand for healthcare services will skyrocket. The shift away from hospitals to other facilities, including the home, will be joined by the same needs that dominated home healthcare in the 1800s: convenience, familiarity, and the presence of family caregivers. For home healthcare providers, helping baby boomers care for their parents—and later, helping "Generation X" take care of the boomers—certainly fuels the engine for continued growth in this sector. This time, however, what goes around, will come around only better. The home will increasingly become the desired care site.

TOMORROW'S HOME

It seems obvious to assert that technological growth will continue to accelerate and provide new levels of productive capacity, consumer convenience, entertainment options, and hopefully, improved quality of life. The expansion of technology should similarly enter and transform the home, including its capacity as a care site. Coincident with the fact that the population's health concerns will elevate in importance (given the number of people reaching older age), the ability to use emerging technologies to benefit their health can be expected to take on a more profound significance.

The connected home can be the fulcrum for the delivery of healthcare services at a level we can only imagine today. Our current arsenal of tools, that includes PCs, fax machines, voicemail, cellular phones, CD-ROMS, and the Internet, will grow exponentially and in new forms to create the real prospect of telemedicine in its most literal sense. Fully wireless communication, comprehensive voice recognition systems, and smaller, smarter devices, all planned and installed in homes as pervasively as television, may become the norm.

Already, the seeds for the required technologies have been planted, and an era of fully distributed computing will blossom in the coming decades. With it, every appliance in the home will leap to attention at the user's command: finding and dialing the number requested, diagnosing the "ping" in the car, displaying the recipe for the evening's meal, deciding which ingredients are missing, and ordering them via instant delivery from the grocer. Even more, each machine would borrow the computing power it needed on a moment-to-moment basis by accessing a wider network via wireless signal, without the annoyance of the endless peripherals, such as those linked to today's desktop PCs. The value of becoming digital will be borne out by the opportunities these technologies provide.

With a fully connected home, it can truly become a primary site for healthcare. Instead of just a family first-aid kit, the home will be equipped with a variety of devices that support diagnosis and treatment of episodic conditions and specific diseases. On-line linkages between the doctor's office and the patient's home will enhance the convenience for both parties and take advantage of technology in the home to help people get well.

All kinds of possibilities emerge: the use of hand-held blood analyzers that provide instant laboratory values; point-of-care diagnostics, including the use of x-rays (or something better) transmitted in real time over a cellular modem; telephonic monitoring devices for cardiac function and blood pressure; easy-to-operate, remote-controlled drug delivery devices and dialysis equipment; instant access to prescribed pharmaceuticals; and virtual reality applications to help caregivers "experience" what their loved one is going through and "know" when they are getting better or worse. The power of technology, if used well, can make a dramatic difference in people's lives and can produce a "smarter" home when it comes to medical care.

WHAT'S HAPPENING TO THE NEIGHBORHOOD?

Medicine is practiced locally; however, it remains incredibly fragmented along the continuum of care . . . even within the local community. This structure leads to inefficiencies and waste, a reduced level of care, and impatience that leads to government intervention. Several attempts to create Community Healthcare Information Networks (CHINS) have failed, largely because of the inability or unwillingness of the industry's trading partners to share data on a large scale.

If the focus shifts, as it must, to the local level and technologies are used to manage high-volume transactions with speed, accuracy, and cost effectiveness, local and regional Community Healthcare Enterprises (CHE) can emerge to realize the dream of a more integrated system.

A CHE is a real-time, multimedia information network, electronically linking and allowing interactive transactions between the primary healthcare trading partners, which includes patients/consumers, providers, employers, payers and government. A CHE can provide competitive advantages in pricing, and managing and providing outcomes, while avoiding the structural pitfalls that belie the system today. Even though a CHE is based on a community level, it can link to other networks, forwarding and retrieving information from outside the local network to anywhere in the world, providing both public and private secured channels.

A CHE can be built by using TCP/IP protocols, developing a series of intranets, linked together around secure access to data repositories. A hospital intranet could connect with step-down facility intranets, and major employer intranets. These in turn would be connected to physician and physician organization intranets, payer intranets, and all be accessible to those at (the connected) home. The ability to interact, to speed the flow of data, to minimize redundancy and to comply with administrative and payment mechanisms, within a local community, will change the way medicine is delivered.

For homebound patients, the "neighborhood" in which care is rendered is similarly changed for the better. The left hand will know what the right hand is doing, and both can be mobilized to assure quality outcomes.

POWER TO THE PEOPLE

Consumer power will exert itself on reimbursement, the delivery systems, technology, and the outcomes related to healthcare. In turn, each of these forces will have a sizable impact on home healthcare.

Asking consumers to take more responsibility for their health brings with it greater obligations for those doing the asking. In this case, employers, providers, and payers—all of whom have interests in reducing costs—will themselves have to be more accountable. Glaring examples of waste, duplication, ineffective record systems, inflated overhead, and confusion will be hard to tolerate at the same time that the system is demanding more from its users.

The interests of maturing baby boomers have turned to asset preservation and family interests. More couples rely on two incomes, probably as many as 80% over the next two decades. At the same time, the definition of *family* is becoming more diverse. Single parents will comprise approximately 40% of the American families with children. The net result is that the traditional caretaker of elderly parents—the "stay-at-home" wife, aunt, or daughter—is a vanishing species. Hence the increased demand for new ways to enable working people to accommodate the needs of children and sick family members. Among the possible solutions is the growing capability to take greater advantage of telecommunications and other technologies.

Consumers have embraced the many easy-to-use medical kits that are bringing laboratory standards into the home, including cholesterol-testing kits, blood pressure monitors, and pregnancy tests. Books, magazines, and CD-ROMS about health are best-sellers. Many types of hospital equipment are now readily available to the private shoppers. Putting these trends together with the spread of computerized communications, one can easily imagine the affluent and "wired" consumer of the next decade, and hence, most everyone soon thereafter, organizing most of his or her medical needs from his or her own homes.

This kind of take-charge attitude bodes well for home healthcare providers. More than other areas of healthcare, home healthcare providers always have relied on patient and family participation in the treatment plan, and they will require even greater participation as more complex services are delivered at home in the future.

There are also pitfalls that come with the expansion of home healthcare technology. It creates an increasing role on patients and their families. For example, patients may suffer if families take on more than they are capable of. Excessive burdens may be placed on caregivers—a disproportionate number of whom are women. It is important to recognize that the worst home is not necessarily better than the best hospital.

What does all this mean for home healthcare? It is entirely possible that home healthcare may eclipse hospital care in the not-so-distant future. At the same time, there is every indication that home healthcare will be called on to invade the arena of long-term care's territory as well. This will present an opportunity for both acute and long-term care organizations to develop home healthcare divisions or to partner with home healthcare providers.

By using common assessment and clinical management tools, such as clinical pathways, physicians will channel qualifying patients who previously would have been hospitalized directly from their offices into home healthcare. Candidates include many patients with pneumonia, pulmonary and infectious diseases, and various chronic cardiovascular and vascular conditions.

WHAT COULD HAPPEN . . .

Everyone has their collective eyes on the future as we enter the new millennium. Technology will no doubt play a significant role as we look out over the next 25 to 50 years. The authors took a leap of faith and suggest the following as possible occurrences:

Home Healthcare Scanners

Home healthcare scanners may enable consumers to safely monitor certain risk factors on a routine basis. Diseases and conditions such as osteoporosis, breast cancer, prostate cancer, cardiovascular disease, headaches, and pregnancy may be easily identified, and the results of "scanned" testing may be automatically transferred to the patients' healthcare team for further evaluation and follow-up as appropriate.

The prospects of such scanning devices rest on the dramatic decrease in size and increase in the complexity of microprocessors that can be used for diagnostic purposes. Further advances in diagnostic tool design and multivariate analyses will improve the likelihood of valid symptom identification and reporting.

Care in the Comfort of Home

The patient is truly the center of the healthcare system. All systems, procedures, scheduling, payments, and continuing care are built around the patient's needs. Diagnostic tools and devices, and telecommunication techniques, enable information about the patient's condition to be available in real time to the appropriate provider of care. Systems of alerts and triage permit immediate attention to those who need it, with the information coming from wherever the patient happens to be. Data systems are robust, integrated and secure, so that there are automatic checks on eligibility and the patient never has to deal with this matter. Similarly, the right provider is made available based on the patient's condition, and that provider has the patient's complete medical history and a personalized guideline for treatment for the patient's specific needs at the time.

Pharmaceuticals may be delivered sooner. Home healthcare equipment may arrive simultaneously, because the agency is also linked into the management of the patient's condition. Payments are handled electronically, through linkages with payers and/or the patient's bank, of course, with a system of checks and balances to monitor corrections. There are no paper or forms. It is all part of the integrated data system, in which the sole objective is for the patient to get better.

Outcome-Based Systems

A consumer revolt against a system that spends 20% or more of the healthcare dollar on administration will significantly reduce the role of middlemen. If data systems are sufficiently linked and automated, home healthcare will assume a more prominent role, which would free up a significant number of dollars now being spent on debt service, physical plant operation, maintenance, and costly infrastructures. The savings would be channeled into more and better treatment systems.

Clinicians will be better able to determine a course of treatment and direct how care can be most effectively rendered. If they are truly supported by the technology, able to effortlessly access broad knowledge bases, and incentivised by the medical outcomes, they can then assume a new level of clinical and fiduciary responsibility that makes everyone a winner.

Information Validation Software

Information validation software is a major application of artificial intelligence that will automatically determine the validity of all health information on the Internet by phrase or statement and provide substantiating research documentation, including the most recent scientific references to verify the accuracy of content. This capability will also extend to consumers' voice statements, including highly specific health questions.

This innovation will enable consumers to avoid wasting time browsing through unnecessary information. We will access answers to questions that in the past took from several minutes or hours to locate. For example, determining what foods are most likely to cause allergies, or for a 58 year old six-foot tall male, what are the normal ranges for body weight, blood pressure, and cholesterol? Answers to simple questions like these will be developed first and followed by more abstract questions, such as, what is the best single approach to self-manage gastroesophageal reflux disease without taking medication?

The interpretation of text involves determining the meanings of words in a particular context and the use of other words that illicit the same meanings. This software will understand complete commands and questions, not just fragments of text. Many years of effort will be required to completely describe health knowledge and map concepts together, from which many new related applications will emerge. Ultimately, clinical problem solving will be an integral part of this software. Providers and consumers will use it to locate and clarify information, ensure informed consent, and make more healthy decisions.

The value of patient empowerment hinges on the validity of the information used. By expediting and validating information retrieval from a common source, consumers and providers will be able to communicate even better.

Global Standardization

The world is becoming a more negotiable space, thanks to new technologies. America is recognized as a leader in the science and technology of medicine, however, many other discoveries are taking place all around the world. Working together with other scientists internationally, there is an opportunity to create a new type of global alliance, one that shares information in an effort to treat and cure disease. This will also provide for leadership that initiates worldwide standards of treatment practice. This Global Care Alliance (GCA) will provide a central point to access information regarding the latest research worldwide.

There would be an international conference to exchange ideas. This conference will be broadcast globally over the Web through telecommunications connectors.

Engineered Food Products

Engineered food products will be available for various diseases and conditions enabling many patients to have more choice without jeopardizing their health. It will improve dietary intake, personal preferences, and quality of life. The impact of culture and diet on health status will be fully defined and modifications will be made in the composition of certain foods to prevent disease and enhance health.

Many dietary practices, particularly in areas where certain foods associated with health problems are locally produced, accessible, and affordable, need not be modified since health risks can be removed from such foods through genetic engineering. This capability will significantly reduce the incidence of coronary heart disease, certain cancers, age onset diabetes, and other conditions associated with eating habits.

Food products will have additives for treating certain diseases. In addition, some foods will be engineered to interact with certain therapeutic agents to both prevent and treat certain diseases and conditions.

Specialized foods engineered to meet the health needs of individuals represent a vast arena of HHT applications that will expand our understanding and use of the relationship of diet to disease prevention, treatment, and health enhancement.

Fad Diets: A Thing of the Past

Total weight management will also be improved through this innovation. Diets created from modified foods used within different cultures, while recognizing personal preferences, will effectively address the lifestyle changes required for weight management.

Tailored diets and related biological programs, responding to the preferences, characteristics, and needs of the each individual will be ordered from the home and delivered by local vendors. Furthermore, these diets will be monitored based on specific individual chemistry levels, such as blood values, hormonal and metabolic indicators.

The vitamin and mineral content of foods will be regulated to the levels that are highly effective in providing essential nutrients for optimum health, and they will be tailored to individual needs. Exercise programs will be created to interface with dietary needs and changed when appropriate.

Home Health Ecosystems

Various diseases and conditions are subject to the impact of the home environment. Among the more obvious environmental home healthcare risks are physical injury, environmental health threats (e.g., radon gas), lack of sunlight, and pollutants in the water and air. The establishment of a home ecosystem specific to the healthcare needs of its residents will contribute significantly to disease management and prevention.

The use of light to treat depression is already established as an effective therapeutic and preventive measure for many patients. Those with mobility problems and the frail elderly, represent special populations for which home health ecosystem modifications will prove effective in reducing morbidity and enhancing quality of life.

Detectors and sensors will assess the status of the home environment and make appropriate adjustments through a computerized control system. Specific environmental healthcare applications will be possible through HHT links between the home and healthcare providers. For example, certain asthma patients will benefit from improvements in the composition of home air.

Eco-Engineers

There will be a new profession borne out of the implementation of home health ecosystems: eco-engineers. Health science engineers will be trained, and specialize in manipulating the entire home environment, as deemed appropriate by health care providers for various diseases and conditions, such as asthma, depression, and allergies. Air quality, composition, light and noise levels, including various methods of stress management, will be among the many controllable elements within the home.

Consumers will be involved in monitoring their environment to achieve a vital balance of elements that make up the home health ecosystem. An understanding of the relationship of the home environment to medical problems and health enhancement will be established and applied through HHT links that will enable modifications conducive to the consumer's health.

Electronic Vision and Hearing Devices

In the future, it is likely that implants will enable those who are blind to see and those who are deaf to hear. Major prerequisites in providing home healthcare are the patient's ability to see or hear. Although various compensatory technologies are available, being able to use one's visual or auditory senses on a relatively normal basis inside and outside of the home has significant advantages in preventing and managing health problems and improving quality of life. The use of HHT applications will assist patients with restored vision or hearing in their transition to a more normal lifestyle in a safe and healthy fashion.

Devices that can be attached to home computer systems will provide ongoing assessments for vision and hearing, as well as other senses and necessary functions. These monitors will communicate via telecommunications with ophthalmologists, audiologists, and ENTs for example who can then make any modifications or change the course of treatment.

Virtual Reality Health Information

Virtual reality technology (VRT) will dramatically facilitate health education by presenting and applying information within simulated life situations conducive to individual decision-making, problem solving, and evaluation. The consequences, whether positive or negative, of those decisions will be played out in a manner that participants will better understand and appreciate the concepts and principles involved. For example, education of the masses to provide cardiopulmonary resuscitation (CPR) will be provided using VRT. Whether or not the trainee saves the simulated victim will be the ultimate test. The management of many health emergencies, in addition to preventive measures, will be enhanced by VRT applications.

Virtual reality therapy will become an adjunct to psychotherapy or drug therapy for many mental disorders. Therapeutic modules will address depression, stress, and anxiety disorders. Emphasis will be placed on coping skills, working from the simple to the complex. Patient evaluation sections will enable patients and healthcare providers to determine the level of progress in VRT-delivered therapy. Providers will be able to refine the patient's treatment plan by shifting VRT therapy to address idiosyncrasies and progress. The modules will also be routinely used for behavioral reinforcement of patients.

Virtual Health Educators

VRT will play a major role in both education and therapy by the year 2050. This will plant the seeds for new professional opportunities. The emerging field will require persons who can write, create, implement, research, and teach in this new milieu. There will be the need for ever-changing lesson materials due to constant new scientific discoveries.

Real-life situations with opportunities to make decisions and experience the consequences will be readily available. Persons will progress through a series of educational or therapeutic scenarios that solicit responses that are immediately evaluated. The educational and therapeutic advantages of this approach to behavior modification is well established by the long history of training aircraft pilots through the use of flight simulators.

These interactive educational programs will be designed to apply information and knowledge, assess learner progress, identify remedial educational needs, and reward the learner. The cognitive, affective, and action domains of the educational process will be combined to establish the virtual reality of life situations. By exploring selected pathways within each scenario, participants will play a major role in health education and training of professionals as well as patient's learning.

Admissions to Health Institutions

For elective admissions, patients will receive a communications device from the healthcare institution. It will have on-screen instructions to facilitate registration and access to the dial-up hospital database/intranet. All necessary pre-admission forms will appear on-screen and are submitted by the patient electronically. The device would permit access to those who could answer questions from the patient or family. This would be possible through the use of e-mail or by telephone.

Access to knowledge databases providing information on clinical guidelines or protocols will offer more opportunities for the patient to understand treatment methodologies and thereby, increase the cooperative effort between patients and their providers.

Robocare

As multiple forms of treatment become available, so do the complexities of care management. These varied options are expected to exacerbate the already growing problem of compliance.

There will be very sophisticated robotics available that will help address this issue especially as it pertains to pharmacology. Currently there is equipment that can dispense medicines in a timely way, however they are still relatively unsophisticated.

These new devices will be multi–task oriented and programmable to the individual. They will not only dispense but will also have sophisticated monitoring mechanisms that connect the consumer to the professional and family caregiver so as to provide information and alert those persons as appropriate.

If you think this one is far off into the future—think again! Currently robotics are used in almost every industry, it's just that we don't notice them. For instance most automakers use robots on the assembly line; the dairy industry uses robots to milk the cows; when you go into cafeteria at work, at the airport or train station you often buy food from an automated vending machine; and yes, the healthcare industry uses this technology in surgery, to assist patients out of bed or into a bathtub, and in artificial limbs.

Longitudinal Health Records

Longitudinal health records (LHRs) will be initiated and maintained by persons from their homes. Since most births occur in hospitals, these sites are readily identifiable as centers where communication devices can be distributed, enabling basic data entry and storage service. An easy-to-read "form" will be filled out before leaving the hospital and will be modified thereafter. The records will be password protected and accessed only by those to whom the patient gives permission. A note will be appended describing the labor and delivery. In time the LHR will begin prior to conception by those pre-planning reproductive events and then the pregnancy will be chronicled, thus providing for future data mining opportunities to correlate pregnancy events with future development.

Adding to this "go forward" process all medical encounters can be a starting point for initiating an LHR. Everyone will be encouraged to begin an LHR at any stage along the life continuum, even those of advanced age.

Electronic Appointments

In the future, people will schedule necessary appointments electronically. Their assessments will precede them to the office, emergency room, or hospital along with the results of whatever has been done during previous encounters, thus eliminating the need for duplicating studies.

Second opinions, consultations, and formal advice will be available to individuals at home from a variety of providers licensed in each state. Easy access to knowledge bases, and decision support systems that can be uniquely responsive to the individual.

Continuing developments in technology will offer some immediate opportunities for preventative and treatment interventions at home to enhance the quality and decrease the cost of care.

CONCLUSION

Clearly, telecommunications currently plays a significant role in home healthcare today. Ambulatory patients are given equipment to wear at home in order to monitor cardiac functions, and they can even send a telephonic message that provides an EKG strip. Recently a respiratory device has become available which monitors oxygen utilization through telecommunication. This enables the care provider immediate access to information about the patient's respiratory therapy.

Audio connections are being combined with video connections to improve the capacity to provide home healthcare. For instance, there are telephone-connected computer systems in use that allow the patients to transfer data to the professional regarding glucose levels and get feedback about their treatment regime including medications, exercise, and diet.

There are electronic health games that are designed specifically for children. This is a chance to teach children about their disease such as asthma, in a way that is interesting to them.

The Internet phone will do much to increase access to information through many avenues. It will assist the consumer, the family member or caregiver and the clinician to interface in real time and provide the needed vehicle to collect and analyze data.

Telephone-video conferencing is increasing the number of on-line home healthcare visits in an effort to more frequently and better monitor a patient's condition. These technological gains will reduce healthcare costs and improve the quality of life for many individuals. This will occur when information is provided to the consumer so that they can act as partner with the professional to better manage their care and reduce emergency room visits and hospital admissions. In addition, this will help curb the skyrocketing costs associated with those who are non-compliant.

Home healthcare telecommunications (HHT) is the present and the future. The savvy providers of healthcare and those companies who manufacture and supply the industry with telecommunications and computer technology are already in discussions and making plans for 2025.

APPENDIX

Resources

American Telemedicine Association

901 15th St. NW
Suite 230
Washington, DC 20005
(202) 408-0677
(202) 408-1134 (fax)
http://www.atmeda.org

Empower Health Corp.

Chairman: C. Everett Koop, MD
Vice Chairman: John Zaccaro
8920 Business Park Drive, Suite 200
Austin, TX 78759
http://www.drkoop.com
http://www.empowerhealth.com

Health Industry Manufacturer's Association

1200 G St. NW
Suite 400
Washington, DC 20005-3814
(202) 783-8700
(202) 783-8750 (fax)
http://www.himanet.com

National Association for Medical Equipment Services

625 Slaters Lane
Suite 200
Alexandria, VA 22314-1171
(703) 836-6263
(703) 836-6730 (fax)
http://www.names.org

National Association for Home Care

228 7th St. SE
Washington, DC 20003
(202) 547-7424
(202) 547-3540 (fax)
http://www.nahc.org

ABOUT THE AUTHORS

Steven Altman, DBA, is President and Chief Operating Officer of Medical Telecommunications Associates, LLC (MTA). MTA specializes in using information technology to provide connectivity solutions and value-added content for all segments of the healthcare industry. The company is based at EC2, The Annenberg Center at the University of Southern California, an entity formed in 1995 to advance multimedia technology development.

From 1992 until joining MTA in 1995, Dr. Altman was president of SynerCo, Inc., a marketing and management consulting firm serving clients in healthcare, financial services, telecommunications, and real estate industries, among others. His engagements included development and management of the Physicians Capital Source Project, a major initiative of the American Medical Association. Physicians Capital Source was designed to assist physicians making the transition to managed care by helping them develop credible business plans and acquiring the needed capital for implementation.

Dr. Altman's business activities followed an academic career that spanned 20 years and included teaching and administrative appointments at four universities. His leadership responsibilities included serving as President of both Texas A&M University, Kingsville, and the University of Central Florida and as Vice President and Provost at Florida International University. Dr. Altman also held appointments as professor of business management and was the recipient of two awards for excellence in teaching. He is the author of 12 books and over 20 articles on management, organization, healthcare, planning, leadership, and education. Along with his professorial duties, he also served as Assistant Dean of the School of Business at the University of Southern California, Chairman of the Management Department, and chief budget and personnel officer at FIU. He has been a frequent speaker at professional organization meetings, a consultant to management, and a neutral arbitrator on the American Arbitration Association panel.

Dr. Altman has served as president of three Chambers of Commerce, reflecting his interests in forging stronger links between the university and the business community. He has been elected to membership in five Honor societies and has received the Freedom Foundation Gold Medal for Economics Education and the Jewish National Fund's Tree of Life Award. Dr. Altman holds a BA in mathematics from UCLA, and MBA and DBA degrees from the University of Southern California.

Steven Altman, DBA
Medical Telecommunications Associates, Inc.
746 W. Adams Blvd.
Los Angeles, CA 90007-2568
(213) 743-1765
e-mail address: *saltman@mdtel.com*
URL: *www.mdtel.com*

Laura Hyatt, RN, BS, CCM, is one of the world's leading experts on healthcare delivery systems. She has been dubbed a "futurist" by the media and professional publications. Focusing on managing change, executive communications, education and strategic planning, her clients include fortune 500 companies as well as not-for-profit corporations, government and academic organizations.

A native of California, she has over 20 years of experience in the healthcare industry including acute care, post-acute care, physician practice and community services. She has extensive knowledge in development, training, program delivery, managed care and strategic planning. Ms. Hyatt has held the title of Vice President of Development and Vice President of Managed Care for both publicly and privately held companies. She developed and directed one of the first specialty medical groups in Los Angeles. During her tenure at *Lifetime Television,* she was a member of the team responsible for creating the "Physician's Journal Update" program.

She served on the Managed Care Planning Subcommittee (part of the President's referendum on healthcare), is a member of the Board of Directors for the Center for Healthy Aging, the Advisory Board for the National Stroke Association, CARF National Advisory Committee, the Board of Directors of The Associates of Santa Monica College, participates on Advisory Panels for the American Nurses Association, the American Association of Respiratory Care, the American College of Health Care Administrators, the National Managed Health Care Congress, was appointed by the Mayor to the L.A. City Council on Aging, and was on the Founding Board of Directors of the National Subacute Care Association. She is often called upon by state and federal administrations to provide expert testimony for healthcare reform. Ms Hyatt also served on an Advisory Group to the Office of the Assistant Secretary for Planning and Evaluation at the Department of Health and Human Services in Washington, D.C., and was appointed to the recent White House Conference on Aging by the President of the United States.

Ms. Hyatt is a featured speaker at national conferences and appears frequently as a guest on television and radio. Her columns appear in *Continuing Care* and *Long Term Care*

Management, and she is on the Editorial Boards of many national publications including *Healthplan Business Advisor, Case
Review, GCM Journal* and the *Reimbursement Bulletin*. Her
first book *Redefining Healthcare* published by McGraw-Hill
reached the "best-sellers" list. Ms Hyatt is a registered nurse, a
certified case manager, and a certified administrator. She has received numerous accolades, most recently she was honored with
the "Woman of Distinction Award" by the NCOA.

HYATT ASSOCIATES
2956 Kelton Avenue
Los Angeles, CA 90064
(310) 474-5676
e-mail address*: surfsup@att.net*

Ronald L. Linder, EdD, MS, is recognized as a leader in the field of healthcare reform and education. He was President of the Alaska Mental Health Association, 1965–1967, while on faculty at Alaska Methodist University. Dr. Linder was a National Science Foundation Post-Doctoral Fellow in Behavioral Research at Stanford University in 1972. His early research and writing in psychopharmacology (1972–1982) earned Dr. Linder the title of "world authority" on phencyclidine (PCP) abuse, according to the *US News and World Report*. He left San Francisco State University in 1974 for a research position at the University of Southern California School of Medicine. From 1978–1985, he directed professional education programming, in the Department of Health Sciences, UCLA Extension, in healthcare management, medicine, nursing, dentistry, and associated health, and he served on faculty in the UCLA School of Public Health. He established the "UCLA Healthcare Administration and Management Certificate Program" in 1980. He directed the "California PCP Training Project" from 1981–1982 and served on the Medical Advisory Committee on drug testing for the 1984 Olympic Games. Dr. Linder also instructed second-year medical students in psychopharmacology between 1983–1990. He worked with leading clinicians and healthcare professionals throughout the United States in the production of over 1,200 continuing education programs for the Hospital Satellite Network for which he achieved ACCME accreditation, from 1985–1989.

Dr. Linder directed the ambulatory care and education initiative in the Veterans Health Administration and its affiliated medical schools throughout the Western United States from 1991–1995. As President of American Medical Productions, he has produced many Telly Ward winning professional and patient education programs from 1995 to the present. Dr. Linder continues to provide expert testimony in federal, criminal, civil, and State Supreme Courts on drug-related cases.

Ronald L. Linder, EdD, MS
American Medical Productions
224 E. Olive Avenue
Burbank, CA 91502
(818) 848-1730

Ronald J. Pion, MD, clinician, educator, and communicator, brings to *Home Healthcare Telecommunications* a unique blend of knowledge, insight and bold vision. He has been involved in the development and production of television, radio, and other interactive electronic programming for healthcare professionals and patients/consumers for more than 25 years. As a teacher, Dr. Pion has been dedicated to facilitating learning on the part of patients and their families, thereby assisting in disease prevention, health promotion, and wellness enhancement through patient empowerment. Following a successful career in academic medicine, serving on the faculties of the University of Washington and the University of Hawaii, Dr. Pion returned to Los Angeles in 1979 to pursue healthcare telecommunications full time.

Dr. Pion hosted his first medical television series in 1968 on Seattle's PBS station and followed this with a health series for children on Seattle's NBC affiliate (KWG-TV). He co-produced and hosted a health-oriented ABC radio series for teenagers and organized the nation's first hospital-based closed-circuit television system for patients at Kapiolani Maternity Medical Center in Honolulu. During the 1970s, Dr. Pion co-developed and hosted a parenting series on Hawaii's PBS station, and he produced patient education videos designed to help document informed consent. He served as medical correspondent for KNBC's *Alive and Well* news feature in Los Angeles (1980) and was the founder of Hospital Satellite Network (HSN) in 1982. HSN designed, produced, and distributed accredited education and training programs. The network became an innovative leader in developing cost-efficient medical video teleconferencing during the 1980s. In 1988 he co-developed and hosted a nationally syndicated daily television series, *Group One Medical,* and hosted disease-management videocassettes targeted to the homecare audience. He was host of *Milestones in Medicine,* a regular Sunday night feature of Lifetime Medical Television during the 1991 and 1992 seasons and recently hosted a new series of videocassettes for patients produced by the Hume Medical Group of Toronto.

Dr. Pion is currently Chairman and CEO of Medical Telecommunications Associates and medical director of Belson-Hanwright Video, Inc. He served on the board of directors of the American Academy of Home Care Physicians (1994–1995) and the Abbey HealthCare Group, Inc. until 1995. He currently serves on the boards of HELP Innovations, Inc., and American Enterprise Solutions, Inc.

Dr. Pion is a graduate of New York University (BA, Phi Beta Kappa) and New York Medical College (MD, Alpha Omega Alpha). He is a clinical professor at the UCLA School of Medicine and a Fellow of the American College of Obstetricians and Gynecologists.

Ronald J. Pion, MD
Medical Telecommunications Associates, Inc.
746 W. Adams Blvd.
Los Angeles, CA 90007-2568
(213) 743-1765
e-mail address: *rpion@mdtel.com*
URL: *www.mdtel.com*

INDEX